thyroz⊘ne

*Real Thyroid
Solutions for
Better Health and
Better Living*

Dr. John A. Robinson
Dr. Cristina Romero-Bosch

ThyroZone: Real Thyroid Solutions for Better Health and Better Living

Published by Wheatmark®
2030 East River Road, Suite 106
Tucson, Arizona 85719 USA
www.wheatmark.com

ISBN: 978-1-62787-489-2 (paperback)
ISBN: 978-1-62787-490-8 (ebook)
LCCN: 2017939209

To the intrepid patient who never settles for less, who is always looking for more, who drives us and every physician to provide real solutions and compassionate relief.

Contents

Section 1

An Introduction to the Thyroid Gland and The ThyroZone® System

Have you ever believed you had a low thyroid problem but the blood test results from your regular doctor always came back normal? Have you ever looked at the list of the symptoms of low thyroid and believed you had many of them, but still could not get the blood test numbers from your regular doctor to confirm it? Maybe you got the diagnosis of low thyroid and took thyroid medication, kept telling your doctor you still had the symptoms related to low thyroid, but were told that your labs were normal, and nothing was done about it? Or maybe your doctor gave you a prescription for some other kind of medication to help with your symptoms, just definitely not an increased dose of your thyroid hormone medication?

What if you could finally get a doctor who listened to you and knew how to effectively diagnose your thyroid problem and give you answers to feeling better right away? What if you had a doctor who could help you get on the most effective thyroid medication dose, despite what a simple blood test result says? What if your metabolism soared, your energy sky-rocketed, your mood improved, and you could finally start losing weight? What if you could feel better now, like you have only imagined?

ThyroZone finally has answers for these questions and more. Since 2006, my wife, Cristina Romero-Bosch and I have researched and developed a system that provides an accurate and scientific diagnosis for thyroid and metabolism disorders. Once provided with the precise dose of natural thyroid hormone your body needs, you will be monitored with care and safety by a unique medical method, unlike anything you have ever experienced before.

The book, *The Hormone Zone: Navigate Metabolism Towards Whole Health Transformation*, covered thyroid health and the entire endocrine system, researched and studied within the context of a holistic and naturopathic viewpoint. This book is designed to focus exclusively on our work with the thyroid, and the unique medical treatment system that was born from that effort: ThyroZone. This book is written in a clear, uncomplicated format. This book is designed for the patient. This book is for you.

To your health,
John A. Robinson, NMD
Cristina Romero-Bosch, NMD

Why ThyroZone?

The Epidemic of Thyroid Disease

An estimated 20 million Americans suffer from hypothyroidism (low thyroid), according to the American Thyroid Association. Other estimates run as high as 60 million, depending on the study criteria used, such as the interpretation of the TSH test values. We tend to agree with the later estimates based on our functional interpretation of thyroid laboratory values and comprehensive view of metabolism and the body. The prevalence rates of hyperthyroidism (high thyroid) and the related autoimmune condition Grave's Disease in the U.S. are about three to four million people.

Thyroid disorders are also eight to 10 times more common in women, and even more common in women over 50 years old, entering menopause. One woman in eight will develop a thyroid disorder during her lifetime.

Most thyroid disorders manifest as hypothyroidism (low thyroid) with the autoimmune condition known as Hashimoto's thyroiditis. In our medical practice, we see men and women with thyroid disorders on a daily basis, coming to see us because they know that something is wrong and that it may be their thyroid. Very often, they find that their instincts are right.

The Epidemic of Inadequate Thyroid Treatment

If a doctor discovers a thyroid condition, particularly the more common hypothyroidism (low thyroid), and prescribes thyroid hormone medication, it will be Synthroid® or the generic form, levothyroxine. In 2015, the name brand hypothyroid drug Synthroid® was the most prescribed drug in the United States, with 21.6 million prescriptions. This does not even include the number of generic prescriptions for levothyroxine.

Taking thyroid hormone medication is called "T4 Mono-therapy." It is this approach of prescribing the singular thyroid hormone levothyroxine (T4), the *inactive* form of thyroid hormone, that is at the heart of why patients very often do not experience relief of their symptoms. The ThyroZone system was created in response to this problem.

What If There Is More?

You've been wondering far too long, "What if there is more? What if I could feel better? I just know it's my thyroid, why doesn't my doctor know it?" So far, you feel you've received no true validation of your symptoms and complaints. You may have wandered out of your doctor's office with a new prescription in your hand that has nothing to do with managing your thyroid symptoms or your metabolism. You are confused, yet certain of your feelings that your thyroid is off or maybe you are not getting enough thyroid medication or, maybe, it could be your other hormones.

ThyroZone offers answers to your questions. Real solutions. Real action. Now!

Your ThyroZone Answers

ThyroZone is a highly developed comprehensive thyroid management system that provides patients with an accurate diagnosis for thyroid disease and effective solutions to deliver real results. One of the most important medical aspects of ThyroZone is the diagnosis it provides you through your metabolic rate, a key measurement that reflects overall health. Through a medically proven system using unique and distinct objective measurements and alternative lab analysis, a potential diagnosis of a thyroid disorder can be achieved where conventional approaches fail.

The other important medical aspect of the ThyroZone system is its treatment process. The first step in treatment seeks to treat and eliminate the causes of the thyroid condition allowing your thyroid and metabolism to function optimally. Secondly, treatment will include the use of multiple nutritional and medical tools. The third step incorporates natural prescription medication in doses that achieve complete symptomatic relief and improve metabolism. The ThyroZone process becomes complete after the comprehensive plan prepared for the patient has addressed all other hormone imbalances. As you can see, there are several steps to the plan.

ThyroZone Treatment Steps

1. Reveal the causes of thyroid hormone imbalance.
2. Treat the causes of the imbalance.
3. Support treatment through nutrition and botanical medicine.
4. Achieve optimized dosing of natural prescription medications.
5. Prepare a plan for comprehensive hormone balance.

Your Thyroid: The Wonder Gland

Before we get started with the ThyroZone system, let's explore some basics about your thyroid gland and its hormones.

Your thyroid gland is one of the most important glands in your body. It secretes a set of hormones that are vital to your entire system. Every cell in your body, head to toe, inside and out, needs thyroid hormone to function properly. When thyroid hormones are not in the correct balance, a person can suffer from multiple symptoms in many different areas. Let's take a closer look at the anatomy and location of the gland in your body to better understand its function.

Thyroid Anatomy

The thyroid gland is a brownish-red gland located at the front of the lower neck, about the level of the thyroid cartilage or Adam's apple, on either side of the trachea or windpipe. The gland may have an H or U shape, formed from two lobes and a connecting piece of thyroid tissue called the isthmus. Each lobe is about five to six cm long (about two and a half to three inches) and weighs about 30 grams in adults. It is usually heavier in women.

The thyroid is composed of two primary cell types: follicular and parafollicular cells, each with its own significant function, explained below.

Follicular Cells

These spherical follicular cells trap iodine from the blood to produce thyroid hormone. Within follicular cells is another feature known as colloid, which stores the materials for thyroid hormone production such as the amino acid tyrosine and a very important thyroid protein called thyroglobulin (TG) that directly participates in the production of thyroid hormone. Thyroglobulin (TG) and thyroid peroxidase (TPO) interact with tyrosine and iodine to start the process of producing thyroid hormones. You will see later on, that the autoimmune condition known as Hashimoto's thyroiditis is caused by your own immune system attacking thyroid gland tissue, particularly the "TG" and the "TPO" which are responsible for making thyroid hormone. When TG and TPO are attacked and become dysfunctional, you do not make thyroid hormone efficiently, causing hypothyroidism (low thyroid). This autoimmune attack can also lead to Grave's disease which leads to hyperthyroidism (high thyroid).

Parafollicular Cells

These thyroid cells are found interspersed within the follicular cells. Parafollicular cells produce calcitonin, which is partially responsible for calcium regulation. Calcitonin helps to shuttle calcium from the blood into your bones. (See below for more information on Calcitonin.) Calcitonin is an often forgotten thyroid hormone that is not usually considered in thyroid disease. The ThyroZone system keeps this hormone in mind, particularly with the use of natural desiccated thyroid hormone medication that actually contains small amounts of naturally occurring calcitonin.

Parathyroid Glands

You have four small bean-sized parathyroid glands that sit within the thyroid gland tissue; there are two parathyroids on each of the two lobes of the thyroid gland. Despite their close proximity to the thyroid gland, the parathyroid glands are distinct glands with their own separate function. These glands secrete parathyroid hormone (PTH), which regulates calcium levels in the blood. In turn calcium controls muscle contractions and many other cellular functions. It is vital that calcium is maintained in very specific levels within the blood and PTH, along with the hormone calcitonin, are responsible for this.

Thyroid Physiology and Your Thyroid Hormones

Now that you know more about the anatomy of the thyroid gland and where it is located in your neck, let's explore the actual hormones that the gland secretes. The interaction of all of your thyroid hormones is a hormone cascade of events that start with the hypothalamus in your brain, stimulating the pituitary gland, then your thyroid gland itself, and finally the target tissues of your body. This is a finely orchestrated process that keeps thyroid hormone levels at normal production rates.

T4 and T3

The primary hormone that is synthesized by the gland is thyroxine (levothyroxine) or T4. It consists of a central tyrosine molecule with four attached iodine molecules, hence its name: T4. Thyroxine is considered a pro-hormone because it is inactive and does not have any direct physiological effect on body cells. Most doctors prescribe a type of synthetic T4 hormone, such as Synthroid® or levothyroxine.

Thyroxine or T4 is converted by the body cells when one iodine molecule is cleaved off, forming triiodothyronine or T3, the active hormone. The T3 that is converted from T4 is what gets into each cell of the body to make it function optimally.

This list describes some of the actions of thyroid hormones in the human body:

- Promote cells to function and develop optimally, vital for normal development in children.
- Assist in bringing sugar (glucose) into the cell, not just insulin.
- Stimulate amino acids from proteins in the diet to transport into the cell, for tissue repair.
- Assist fats to be metabolized, assisting in weight loss.
- Enhance vitamin metabolism, to get more out of your nutrition and supplements.
- Improve the liver's ability to make sugar (glucose) and to

eliminate excess cholesterol, bringing down cholesterol levels in the blood.

- Stimulate neurochemicals in the brain such as serotonin, dopamine and norepinephrine, which enhance and regulate mood as well as stimulate the natural production of human growth hormone.
- Decrease substance P, a molecule in the body associated with increased pain sensation.
- Increase basal (resting) metabolic rate, giving you energy.
- Increase recovery rate from exercise.
- Stimulate heart tissue and enhances cardiac output.
- Maintain fertility and enable pregnancy. Note: One of the most important considerations in infertility is optimal thyroid function.

Calcitonin

Calcitonin acts to reduce blood calcium, opposing the effects of parathyroid hormone (PTH), which increases blood calcium levels. Calcitonin prevents bone breakdown and promotes excretion of calcium through the kidneys. Most doctors treating patients for thyroid disease, particularly hypothyroidism (low thyroid), do not consider this hormone. When you take the medication levothyroxine (T4), then you do not receive the benefits of calcitonin. However, natural desiccated thyroid hormone, such as Nature Throid®, contains small amounts of calcitonin. It is interesting to note that estrogen therapy in menopausal women helps to promote calcitonin production, which helps to lower osteoporosis risk.

In Summary

Thyroid hormone comes down to one concept: metabolism. Hormonal health, in general, relates back to optimal metabolism. If the metabolism within a cell or body organ is diminished, then the health of that cell or organ is diminished, leading to a multitude of problems. The ThyroZone system is designed to bring that metabolism back online and keep it there!

3

Diseases of the Thyroid Gland

Thyroid disease presents in epidemic proportions. According the American Thyroid Association, in the United States, there are over 20 million people with diagnosed thyroid disorder, or about one in 13. Another 13 million people suffer from an undiagnosed thyroid disorder, or one in 20. Of these estimates, about 75 percent of the thyroid disorders are due to hypothyroidism (low thyroid). Extrapolated data would estimate approximately 518 million people worldwide, or about 7.5 percent of the world population, are suffering with some form of thyroid disorder.

There are several disorders related to the thyroid gland. In this chapter, you will begin to understand the main conditions related to the thyroid gland including causes and the inevitable results.

Hypothyroidism

This is the most common form of thyroid disease. Hypothyroidism refers to a low functioning or underactive thyroid gland. In hypothyroidism there is too little thyroid hormone available to the body to make it operate normally. As already mentioned, in the United States alone, there is a massive epidemic of hypothyroidism with estimates of 20 million sufferers. Many are diagnosed but still suffer from the symptoms because of inadequate comprehensive treatment. But many do not know they have the condition and remain undiagnosed and untreated.

The main result of hypothyroidism is a lowered metabolic rate with its consequent array of varied symptoms and problems affecting the entire body. In Chapter 5 there is a detailed questionnaire that lists many of the symptoms related to hypothyroidism. The main take home message right now is that your thyroid governs metabolism. And when your metabolism is slow, as it is in hypothyroidism, you suffer. Some of the key symptoms of hypothyroidism are fatigue, weight gain, hair loss, dry skin, digestive disturbances, constipation, anxiety, depression, and joint pain, to name just a few.

Hashimoto's Thyroiditis

Hashimoto's thyroiditis is an autoimmune condition. Autoimmunity refers to the process where the immune system, which helps fight disease in the body, is triggered by an environmental or genetic cause to attack certain body cells or tissue. In the case of Hashimoto's thyroiditis, there is an immune attack on the thyroid gland that leads to inflammation, destruction of thyroid cells, and inevitable low thyroid function. Hashimoto's thyroid-itis is the number one reason we see low thyroid conditions in the U.S. population.

If someone has an underactive thyroid gland caused by Hashimoto's thyroiditis, then they have all of the potential symptoms of hypothyroidism (low thyroid) along with some additional symptoms and problems associated with the auto-immune process. Some of these additional symptoms can be an enlarged thyroid (goiter) that becomes swollen and irritated in a random fashion, tongue swelling, hoarseness, fever, and agita-tion. Patients will experience a "Hashimoto's Flare" which means that symptoms can become exacerbated very quickly in a seem-ingly random fashion.

What Causes Hypothyroidism and Hashimoto's Thyroiditis?

There are several causes for both hypothyroidism (low thyroid) and Hashimoto's thyroiditis.

Age and Gender: As you age, the incidence of developing hypothyroidism (low thyroid) and Hashimoto's greatly increases, particularly over the age of 50. And women are eight to 10 times more likely to develop these issues than men.

Nutritional deficiencies: A lack of adequate calories is often overlooked. But even more prevalent is the excessive empty calories that are devoid of fat soluble vitamins such as A, D, E, and K, all important for thyroid function and metabolism. Addi-tionally, and even more important, is the lack of minerals includ-ing the most important, iodine.

Gluten and Wheat Intolerance: One of the most common reasons that lead to Hashimoto's is the consumption of wheat and gluten. Because gluten is an allergen to so many people, it reacts negatively with the thyroid gland, creating an autoimmune reaction.

Genetic Factors: The odds of having hypothyroidism are higher if a family member has the condition. Certain genetic factors will increase the risk of developing either hypothyroidism (low thyroid) or hyperthyroidism (high thyroid).

Endocrine Disruptors Chemicals: These are chemicals that can disrupt the normal function of any gland that secretes hormones, including the thyroid gland. There are over 150 different chemicals that are known to affect thyroid gland function. Some of these include pesticides used in conventionally grown produce and BPA found in plastics.

Stress: Mental and emotional stress impacts the function of the thyroid gland, often leading to low thyroid function and autoimmune reactions.

Overactive Immune Reactions: Both viral and bacterial infections can create a large stress on the immune system, leading to autoimmune reactions such as Hashimoto's. Also, if you already have a diagnosis of another autoimmune condition such as Rheumatoid Arthritis (RA), lupus, Crohn's disease, or Multiple Sclerosis (MS), this increases your risk of having Hashimoto's.

Other Hormone Imbalances: One of the most common reasons to develop hypothyroidism (low thyroid) is due to menopause. As both estrogen and testosterone decline, the function of the thyroid often becomes stressed and leads to low functioning.

Hyperthyroidism

This is an overactive thyroid. It results from the thyroid gland secreting too much thyroid hormone. All of the body cells become

over-stimulated and hyperactive. This can be a more serious condition due to the stimulation of thyroid hormone to the heart.

The main result of hyperthyroidism (high thyroid) is an overactive metabolism. In Chapter 5, there is a detailed questionnaire
that will help to determine if you have the disease. Some of the
most obvious symptoms would be an elevated heart rate, elevated
blood pressure, shaking and tremors in your hands and body,
excessive heat and sweating, agitation, anxiety, rapid weight loss,
and muscle weakness. *Please note: If you believe you are suffering
from hyperthyroidism, seek medical attention immediately.*

Grave's Disease

Grave's disease is the most common cause of hyperthyroidism in the United States. This is an autoimmune condition that
causes the elevated function of the thyroid gland resulting in
high levels of thyroid hormone. Where Hashimoto's means you
have an underactive thyroid, Grave's disease means an overactive
condition with your thyroid gland. But both are autoimmune in
nature.

What Causes Hyperthyroidism and Grave's Disease?

All of the same potential causes of hypothyroidism (low
thyroid) and Hashimoto's thyroiditis will also influence the
development of hyperthyroidism (high thyroid) and Grave's
disease, including age and gender, nutritional deficiencies,
gluten and wheat intolerance, genetic factors, endocrine disruptors chemicals, stress, overactive immune reactions, and other
hormone imbalances. One important factor that contributes to
hyperthyroidism is cigarette smoking. The chemicals in tobacco

smoke can cause hypothyroidism (low thyroid) but the association tends towards causing hyperthyroidism (high thyroid).

Benign Conditions: Thyroid Nodules and Goiter

Some conditions of the thyroid gland are relatively common and benign, such as thyroid nodules, and do not cause any immediate threat. But common does not mean normal! Sometimes, patients are made to feel that "common" is "normal." On the other hand, most benign conditions are just that, benign, not something to cause alarm. Nevertheless, you and your doctor must be vigilant to the *causes* of these conditions and understand how to best prevent them by readjusting your environment in ways that promote and sustain health. These benign conditions are subtle warning signs that something is going on with the thyroid gland and the environment in which it exists. While conventional medical approaches evaluate for the presence of disease, there is no real consideration for why benign conditions occur. The ThyroZone system seeks to help you understand benign conditions while creating a healthier thyroid environment.

Thyroid Nodules

Thyroid nodules are an abnormal growth of thyroid cells that form a lump within the thyroid gland. In the U.S., the prevalence of thyroid nodules is approximately four to seven percent of the population. In order to diagnose and treat thyroid cancer at the earliest stage, all thyroid nodules need some type of evaluation. The basic form of evaluation is to perform a thyroid ultrasound, a simple, noninvasive diagnostic imaging of the thyroid gland. If a thyroid nodule is very small, under 1.0 to 1.5 cm, then the typical approach is to monitor the growth of the nodule over time. If it is greater than 1 or 1.5 cm, then the typical approach is to perform a thyroid biopsy using a technique called Fine Needle Aspiration (FNA). Using a very fine biopsy needle, a small sample is taken from the nodule and the cells are examined for potential thyroid cancer. About 80-95 percent of thyroid nodules are benign (noncancerous), which means five to 20 percent contain thyroid cancer.

Since most thyroid nodules are benign, they are harmless. However, basic thyroid blood work will determine if there is an immediate problem. An examiner or the patient cannot even feel most thyroid nodules. However, sometimes they can. Occasionally, some thyroid nodules are large enough and positioned in such a way where they obstruct swallowing or cause some discomfort with swallowing. If the nodule presents in this way, then surgical removal may be needed. But again, most people have no difficulty with benign thyroid nodules.

Goiter

This is a condition that leads to an enlargement of the thyroid gland. The amount of thyroid hormone from the thyroid gland may still be within normal levels, but there is still dysfunction within the gland itself. This is usually a sign that something else is going on in the body that is leading to the goiter. Usually the condition is benign and causes very few issues. Basic blood work will determine if the gland is either over or under functioning. However, when goiter is very large, it can be very painful and can obstruct swallowing and neck movement.

What Causes Thyroid Nodules and Goiter?

Iodine Deficiency: Worldwide, iodine deficiency is the main cause of goiter. A very large percentage of people in the U.S. are deficient in iodine. The conventional view is that we have plenty of iodine in the U.S., but this is not accurate for many reasons. One of the main reasons is that nutritional advice is based on the absolute minimum levels to sustain some level of function, and does not take into account the goal of health optimization as well as other factors that could be continually depleting a nutrient such as iodine.

When iodine is deficient, thyroid nodules, goiter, and other benign masses are more likely to develop. Iodine deficiency causes something called "hyperplasia" which is an increased number of cells in an area, like the thyroid gland. This hyperplasia leads to thyroid nodules.

Iodine deficiency also causes something called "hypertrophy" which is an enlargement of existing cells, leading to thyroid goiter.

Hashimoto's Thyroiditis: This autoimmune thyroid condition leads to an increased risk of goiter and thyroid nodules. If there is an active autoimmune process happening within the thyroid gland, then there is a higher risk of swelling, goiter, and thyroid nodules.

Neck Radiation: Receiving radiation therapy or testing in the neck area increase the risk of having a thyroid nodule by 16-31 percent.

Thyroid Cancer

Thyroid cancer is the most common endocrine cancer comprising 1.0-1.5 percent of all new cancers diagnosed each year in the U.S., and its worldwide incidence has continuously increased since the 1980s. However, fewer than 2,000 American patients die of thyroid cancer annually. In 2013 over 630,000 patients were living with thyroid cancer in the states.

Females are more likely to have thyroid cancer at a ratio of 3:1. Thyroid cancer can occur at any age, but it is most common after age 30. There are several types of thyroid cancer, but we will focus on three main types, papillary, follicular, and medullary thyroid cancer.

Papillary Thyroid Cancer: This is the most common type of thyroid cancer, accounting for about 80 percent of all thyroid cancer cases. Papillary carcinomas develop from thyroid follicular cells and tend to be slow growing. It has an extremely excellent prognosis and the likelihood of a papillary thyroid carcinoma (tumor) spreading and leading to death is very low. The cure rate for this type of cancer is nearly 100 percent.

Follicular Thyroid Cancer: This is the second most common type of thyroid cancer, accounting for 10-15 percent of cases. It develops in the thyroid hormone producing follicles of thyroid gland. It has a very good prognosis at a cure rate of about 95 percent, slightly lower than papillary cancer. Follicular carcinomas do not usually spread, but they are more likely than papillary cancers to spread to other organs, like the bones or lungs.

Medullary Thyroid Cancer: This cancer develops from C cells in the thyroid gland, cells responsible for making the hormone calcitonin, and is more aggressive than papillary or follicular cancers. About four percent of thyroid cancers are medullary thyroid cancer. Spreading to lymph nodes and other organs, known as metastasis, is at a higher risk. High levels of calcitonin and carcinoembryonic antigen (CEA) can be detected by blood tests helping to differentiate this type of thyroid cancer.

How Do I Detect Thyroid Cancer?

Usually there are not any major symptoms related specifically to thyroid cancer. However, you may be developing the signs and symptoms of either hypothyroidism (low thyroid) or hyperthyroidism (high thyroid) which then leads to getting basic screening. Screening leads to a proper diagnosis.

Blood work can be helpful and is sometimes the first step to determining if thyroid cancer is present. Elevated thyroid antibodies, such as Anti-TPO and Anti-TG, accompanied with any type of neck swelling should be followed up with a thyroid ultrasound. The thyroid ultrasound will help to determine the size of the gland and if there are any large thyroid nodules needing further follow up. Only about one in 10 thyroid nodules have cancer. But if the nodule is large enough a biopsy will be performed. Once the biopsy has been analyzed, then the potential of thyroid cancer can be determined.

The type of thyroid cancer determines the specific course of treatment. But in all types of thyroid cancer, initial treatment includes the partial or total surgical removal of the thyroid, followed by conventional approaches such as chemotherapy if the cancer is aggressive or has spread. After surgery, the usual course of treatment includes hormone replacement medication. At this point, the ThyroZone system is capable of providing the most favorable thyroid hormone treatment and monitoring.

What Causes Thyroid Cancer?

There are several causes for thyroid cancer, most of which can be avoided.

Genetic Risks: If your mother or father had thyroid cancer, your risk is higher.

Iodine Deficiency: This is a common nutrient related to thyroid cancer in general, specifically follicular thyroid cancer.

Radiation Exposure: Years after the Chernobyl nuclear power plant incident in 1986 and even more recently with the Fukushima disaster in 2011, we continually understand the devastating effects of radiation on the thyroid gland leading to an increased risk for goiter (enlarged thyroid), thyroid dysfunction such as hypothyroidism (low thyroid) and hyperthyroidism (high thyroid), and thyroid cancer.

Environmental Toxins: Multiple studies show the correlation of Endocrine Disruptor Chemicals (EDCs) on the thyroid gland. Although at the present time, there is no documented evidence that shows a direct correlation between these chemicals and thyroid cancer, avoiding using products with EDCs is a good idea.

The Complete ThyroZone System

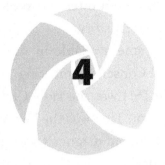

The Science and History

The ThyroZone system was designed to answer questions for the many people suffering from thyroid disease, and provide a comprehensive system beyond the typical conventional medical approach. The ThyroZone system is based on current thyroid science as well as the forgotten and overlooked approaches to comprehensive and rational thyroid care. Historically, thyroid disease, particularly hypothyroidism (low thyroid), was handled rather easily, with very excellent results. Then conventional medicine forgot some things and left some good things behind to embrace the new.

And it wasn't all good.

When you go to your regular doctor, your gynecologist, your internist, even your endocrinologist, they will rely mostly on the blood test called the Thyroid Stimulating Hormone, or TSH. You have likely seen this test before. It is used as the most basic routine test, and it is also used as the most "specific" thyroid test by most doctors; including the endocrinologist.

We are here to say that for the most part, the TSH is a faulty and limited test at best, and often a complete waste of time at worst. Let's explore some history.

The TSH test became available in the early 1970s. At the 1973 Thyroidologists' Consensus meeting in the United States, they agreed that the TSH was the Holy Grail of thyroid disease diagnosis and treatment. That was the beginning of the end of a rational approach to thyroid diagnosis and treatment, and it led to the dilemma of suffering patients we have today. Patients were no longer being helped by doctors who were examining them and considering the typical signs and symptoms of thyroid disease. Instead, they were relying on their new clinical best friend, the TSH. Doctors were now diagnosing low thyroid conditions solely based on TSH results and not on patient history, symptoms and physical examination

Doctors would proclaim it was not a thyroid problem, even though it looked like it clinically, because the TSH was normal.

Patients were feeling horrible and new diseases, traditionally related to low thyroid disease, were emerging. By 1980, the conditions of Chronic Fatigue Syndrome and Fibromyalgia were "discovered." Chronic fatigue and fibromyalgia are conditions that are almost always simply related to low thyroid functioning. The symptoms are essentially the same for both conditions.

Before 1973, physicians would have seen the signs and symptoms of chronic fatigue and fibromyalgia early on and simply treated the patient with thyroid hormone to solve the problem. Hence, no official name for the diseases was needed. But there is a need now because most patients who have low thyroid hormone conditions are not quickly identified because the coveted TSH value is normal. Thus the patient is left to suffer and fully develop disease.

Unfortunately, long-standing chronic fatigue and fibromyalgia are conditions very challenging to reverse if the patient has not been properly treated with thyroid hormone therapy. But challenging does not mean impossible, so there is always hope.

Other conditions like elevated cholesterol, heart disease, depression and other psychiatric disorders, gastrointestinal disorders, and many others are all related to low thyroid disease. These conditions have become more prevalent as the TSH dictated thyroid diagnosis. It is an unfortunate mistake that conventional medicine and endocrinology continue to rely simply on TSH results, not obvious symptoms and patient reporting, to diagnose thyroid disease. More on the TSH later and how the ThyroZone system interprets it...and then goes beyond it.

The Science and History of Thyroid Disease and Treatment

ThyroZone is based on the science and medical traditions that have evolved from the beginning of thyroid disease medical diagnosis and treatment. When Dr. Romero-Bosch and I first began exploration into thyroid science and treatment in 2006, we quickly learned that the best approaches to thyroid hormone management were the methods used prior to the invention of the TSH in the early 1970s.

Before that time, doctors would utilize rational investigative and diagnostic examinations directly on and with the patient. It was not simply a blood test. It was much more. At that time, all doctors, conventional and naturopathic, were trained to use the art of physical examination and measurement. They would take the time to see the patient's world through the art of investigative conversation. They would put their hands on the patient to properly examine them, to better see the large picture. Not inconsequently, this is exactly how thyroid disease diagnosis and treatment was done since the late 1800's, nearly 100 years before the invention of the TSH.

Of course, thyroid patients faired far better then, feeling relief from the thyroid disease, particularly low thyroid. The ThyroZone system is doing just that. It is conserving proven thyroid diagnostic methods all within the cutting-edge backdrop of newer science and technology, to form a complete hormone picture.

Here is a great quote from a world famous endocrinologist Sir R.I.S. Bayliss. He worked as the consultant endocrinologist at Lister Hospital in London, England, was knighted and worked with the royal family. In 1971, in his speech at the Medical Society's Transactions, he answered how to best determine if a patient had adequate thyroid hormone.

> "I am often asked how the correct dose of [thyroid hormone medication] is determined. The answer is clinically by the patient's pulse rate, his sense of wellbeing, the texture of his skin, his tolerance of cold, his bowel function, and **the speed with which his deep tendon reflexes relax.**" (Emphasis added.)

Sir Bayliss told us that the best way to determine thyroid hormone status is how the body is functioning and responding to the direct effects of thyroid hormone. He understood that your body will largely tell you where the dose should be or if thyroid hormone replacement is needed at all. Note that he said nothing of a blood test. At the time, there were some basic labs (not the TSH), but they were not as useful or as easy as simply examining the patient.

Why would the body be able to tell so much about its thyroid gland? Understand that only 18 percent of the thyroid hormones in your body can be found in the blood, while 75 percent can be found in the muscles, skin and brain. Most of the thyroid hormone in your body is in your tissues. How your body is working tells the biggest story. The ThyroZone system helps to reveal this intimate story for the doctor and leads the patient to getting the thyroid hormone they need.

Are thyroid tests worthless? No. Definitely not. We believe in not throwing the baby out with bath water. But like any blood test, we need to examine it within the context of the clinical picture; how a patient is physically, emotionally, and psychologically presenting. Sir Bayliss also wrote,

> *"The amount of* [thyroid hormone] *replacement prescribed seems to be a hit-and-miss business, the dosage being based neither on careful clinical assessment nor on laboratory tests.... Certainly it is my experience that patients feel at their best when the free thyroxine level is towards the upper end of the reference range or marginally above it and the TSH towards the lower limit of the normal range."* "

Practically all of our patients have high end T4 values and low end TSH values. In fact, that is the easy part of how the ThyroZone system doses thyroid hormone medication. The more intricate nature of the ThyroZone system is how to properly examine the patient's physical signs and symptoms, quantify them, monitor them, then relate all of this to the other hormones in their body, and ultimately translate this to an optimal thyroid hormone dose. Most doctors simply do not want to do this with thyroid hormone diagnosis and treatment. However, we do it...for you.

What you will find in the next chapters are the full Thyro-Zone system. Now that you have some historical background, you are ready to delve into the process of determining if you have a thyroid condition, developing a comprehensive treatment plan, and accurately monitoring your progress over time.

You are ready to discover your ThyroZone.

Your Personal Diagnosis

Your personal diagnosis determines aspects about your thyroid gland, your metabolic rate, and overall hormonal picture. The most common thyroid problem is hypothyroidism (low thyroid), and that is the focus of the initial diagnosis of Thyro-Zone. However, you will be screened for hyperthyroidism (high thyroid) too.

Step 1: Basic Screening

ThyroZone starts with a basic (but thorough) clinical, research-proven questionnaire for you to answer about your health. It includes questions that will reveal symptoms of low metabolism and conditions known to be related to hypothyroidism (low thyroid). We start with screening for hypothyroidism because it is the most common condition.

When you come to the office, you will report your physical

signs and symptoms by completing clinical questionnaires. During your visit with the doctor and physical examination, we will use the questionnaires as assessment tools to measure your responses and establish a baseline diagnosis. Reviewing your responses also helps identify any possible issues, and lets you know what to expect in the future.

HYPOTHYROID SYMPTOM QUESTIONNAIRE

Please rank each symptom on the space to the left using numbers from 0 to 5.

0 = none, 1 = very mild, 2 = mild, 3 = moderate, 4 = severe, 5 = very severe.

Which of the following symptoms apply to you at this time?

Dermatological

Dry skin	__/5
Course skin	__/5
Itchy skin	__/5
Dry, coarse hair	__/5
Thinning/loss of hair	__/5
Thinning eyebrows	__/5
Brittle or ridges on nails	__/5
Excess wax in ears	__/5
Decreased sweat	__/5
Paleness of skin or lips	__/5
TOTAL	__/50

Metabolic

Lethargy (low energy)	__/5
Sensation of cold	__/5

Heat intolerance (not hot flashes)	__/5
Slow speech (not memory)	__/5
Weight gain with little food intake	__/5
Lack of appetite	__/5
Lack of libido	__/5
TOTAL	__/35

Dryness (also known as sicca)

Dry eyes	__/5
Dry skin	__/5
Dry mouth	__/5
Dry nose	__/5
Dry sinuses	__/5
Dry vagina	__/5
TOTAL	__/30

Gastrointestinal

Constipation	__/5
Diarrhea	__/5
Irritable bowel syndrome	__/5
GERD (reflux disease)	__/5
TOTAL	__/20

Reproductive

Delayed menstrual flow	__/5
Excessive menstrual flow	__/5
Painful menses	__/5
Impotence (men only)	__/5
TOTAL	__/15

Mental/Emotional Well-being

Depression	__/5
Irritability/mood swings	__/5

Nervousness   __/5
Anxiety   __/5
Impaired memory   __/5
Impaired focus   __/5

TOTAL   __/30

Cardiovascular/Respiratory

Chest pain   __/5
Palpitations   __/5
Atrial fibrillation   __/5
Chronic cough of <u>unknown reason</u>   __/5
Airflow obstruction (non smokers)   __/5
Shortness of breath on physical exertion   __/5
Shortness of breath in general   __/5

TOTAL   __/30

Swelling (edema)

Swollen ankles   __/5
Swollen wrists   __/5
Swollen eyelids   __/5
Swollen, thick tongue   __/5
Swollen face   __/5

TOTAL   __/25

Musculoskeletal

Muscle weakness   __/5
Unexplained tingling or numbness   __/5
Body aches   __/5
Muscle pain   __/5
Joint pain   __/5
Carpal tunnel syndrome   __/5
Plantar fasciitis   __/5

TOTAL   __/35

Sleep

Difficulty getting to sleep	__/5
Difficulty staying asleep	__/5
Wake unrefreshed	__/5
Sleep apnea	__/5
Snoring	__/5
TOTAL	__/25

Scoring: If you score 50 percent or higher in most categories, there is a high likelihood of hypothyroidism (low thyroid and low metabolism).

Step 2: Determining Goiter

During your physical exam, the first step will be to determine if you have an enlargement of your thyroid gland (goiter), and if necessary, you will be referred to have a thyroid ultrasound. The ultrasound will provide a more accurate measurement and classification of your thyroid gland to determine diagnosis and treatment.

World Health Organization (WHO) Classification of Goiter

Grade 0 - No goiter presence is found (the thyroid is impalpable and invisible).

Grade 1 - Neck thickening is present as a result of enlarged thyroid, palpable however, not visible in normal position of the neck; the thickened mass moves upwards during swallowing. Grade 1 includes also nodular goiter if thyroid enlargement remains invisible.

Grade 2 - Neck swelling, visible when neck is in normal position, corresponding to enlarged thyroid detected on palpation.

Step 3: Confirming the Diagnosis: Low or High Thyroid?

If hypothyroidism (low thyroid) is suspected based on the initial thyroid questionnaire and intake information, then the next step is to perform a detailed exam using Zulewski's Clinical Score for hypothyroidism. This tool is a research-based questionnaire proven to aid in the diagnosis of hypothyroidism (low thyroid). A score greater than five points defines hypothyroidism (low thyroid), while a score of zero to two points defines euthyroidism (normal thyroid).

Symptoms are conditions reported by the patient. Physical signs are measurable and directly observable by the examiner. However, a patient may be able to help determine physical signs also.

ZULEWSKI'S CLINICAL SCORE FOR HYPOTHYROIDISM

Symptoms	Symptom Description	Present	Absent
Diminished sweating	Not sweating in a warm room or on a hot summer day when others do	1	0
Hoarseness	Speaking or singing voice	1	0
Paraesthesia	Subjective sensation of tingling or numbness	1	0
Dry skin	Dryness of skin, noticed spontaneously, requiring treatment	1	0
Constipation	Bowel habit, use of laxative	1	0
Impairment of hearing	Progressive impairment of hearing	1	0
Weight increase	Recorded weight increase, tightness of clothes	1	0

Physical Signs	Sign Description	Present	Absent
Slow movements	Observe patient's movements during exam	1	0
Delayed ankle reflex	Observe (measure: ThyroFlex®) the relaxation of the reflex	1	0
Coarse skin	Examine hands, forearms, elbow for roughness and thickening of skin	1	0
Periorbital puffiness	This should obscure the curve of the malar bone (outer upper cheek/eye bone)	1	0
Cold skin	Compare temperature of hand with examiner's	1	0
SUM OF ALL ___/ 12			

Scoring for the Zulewski's Clinical Score for Hypothyroidism: A score of five or above out of 12 strongly suggests that you may have hypothyroidism (low thyroid).

Wayne's Hyperthyroid Index for Hyperthyroidism

You will also go through an exam using the Wayne's Index for Hyperthyroidism (high thyroid). This research-based index explores the possible signs and symptoms for the diagnosis of hyperthyroidism (high thyroid and elevated metabolism). Most patients will present with hypothyroidism (low thyroid) and a smaller percentage will have hyperthyroidism (high thyroid). Wayne's Index will help to determine if your metabolism is elevated and you have hyperthyroidism (high thyroid).

This exam process will often be used to monitor those patients taking thyroid hormone medication to ensure safety and the proper dose. Lab work alone will not be able to determine if you are or are not on too much thyroid medication. The ThyroZone process uses physical signs and symptoms you report about your body to understand where your thyroid hormone dose should be. Much of the following may be unfamiliar, but can be useful for your doctor.

Symptoms of recent onset and/or increased severity	Score	Signs	Present	Absent
Dyspnea on effect (exertion)	+1	Palpable thyroid	+3	-3
Palpitations	+2	Bruit over thyroid	+2	-2
Tiredness	+2	Exopthalmos	+2	-2
Preference for heat	-5	Lid retraction	+2	-
Excessive sweating	+3	Hyperkinesis	+4	-2
Nervousness	+2	Hands hot	+2	-2
Appetite: increased	+3	Hands moist	+1	-1
Appetite: decreased	-3	Pulse rate: < 90	-3	-
Weight increased	-3	Pulse rate: > 90	+3	-
Weight decreased	+3	Atrial fibrillation	+4	-
TOTAL SCORE:				

A score greater than 19 implies toxic hyperthyroidism, while a score less than 11 implies euthyroidism (normal thyroid and metabolism). A score between 11 and 19 is equivocal (uncertain), but helps to guide towards a diagnosis.

RELATED CONDITIONS QUESTIONNAIRE

Do you have either a current or past medical diagnosis of any of the following conditions? Answer Yes or No

Cardiovascular disease	Yes	No
Hypertension	Yes	No

High cholesterol	Yes	No
Infertility/Multiple miscarriage	Yes	No
Anemia	Yes	No
Hypothyroidism	Yes	No
Thyroid nodules	Yes	No
Goiter (enlarged thyroid)	Yes	No
Hashimoto's thyroiditis	Yes	No
Fibromyalgia	Yes	No
Frozen shoulder	Yes	No
Chronic Fatigue Syndrome	Yes	No
Adrenal dysfunction	Yes	No
Addison's disease	Yes	No
Cushing's disease	Yes	No
Lupus	Yes	No
Diabetes type I	Yes	No
Insulin Resistance	Yes	No
Celiac disease	Yes	No
Gluten and/or wheat intolerance	Yes	No
Multiple Sclerosis	Yes	No
Rheumatoid Arthritis	Yes	No
Sjogren's disease	Yes	No
Positive ANA blood test	Yes	No
Polycystic Ovarian Syndrome	Yes	No
Fibrocystic breasts/dense breasts	Yes	No
Currently taking lithium or amiodarone (Cordarone®)	Yes	No
Nonalcoholic fatty liver disease	Yes	No
Dysfunctional uterine bleeding	Yes	No
Amenorrhea (lack of menstrual periods)	Yes	No
Hyponatremia (low blood sodium)	Yes	No
Restless Leg Syndrome	Yes	No
Raynaud's phenomena	Yes	No
Pericarditis	Yes	No
Rhabdomyolysis	Yes	No

Sleep Apnea	Yes	No
Prolactinoma (pituitary tumor)	Yes	No
Psychiatric issues	Yes	No
Bipolar disease	Yes	No

Note: If you have even one of these conditions, it increases the likelihood of having a thyroid condition.

Step 4: A Functional Analysis of Blood Work

Thyroid blood work is probably the most misunderstood of laboratory analyses. The ThyroZone system helps to make this much clearer and more effective. The first step in making thyroid blood work more effective is to understand that thyroid blood work really is NOT that effective!

That may seem strange.

However, when we realize that blood work of any kind, particularly thyroid blood work, is limited in what it can perfectly diagnose then we can move forward and use it correctly. Up to this point, your regular doctors thought of the thyroid labs as the *best* way to diagnose and treat your thyroid and metabolism. For most of you, this does not mean the best situation.

Let's step out of that box together.

The second step is to understand how to interpret the labs and the ranges. It is important to note that thyroid labs are not without merit or usefulness. On the contrary, when placed in the proper context of their fallibility and viewed with a keen eye, they can be helpful in the larger picture of diagnosis and monitoring. When thyroid lab values are looked at a little differently, it can help to diagnose and treat thyroid conditions more accurately than the traditional conventional approach.

The ThyroZone system uses the following thyroid blood tests and predictive ranges:

TSH (Thyroid Stimulating Hormone): This is one of the most confusing tests for patients and doctors alike. TSH is like an email message from your pituitary in your brain that is sent down to your thyroid gland to "stimulate" it to make thyroid hormones such as T4 and T3. If you have an excess of emails coming from your brain, it is because it is trying to scream at a gland that is not producing enough hormones. The higher your TSH value above the optimal range, the lower your overall thyroid function.

Standard Range: 0.45 to 4.5 uIU/mL

Optimal Range BEFORE DIAGNOSIS: 0.3 to 2.0 uIU/mL

Total T3: This is the most active form of thyroid hormone coming from the thyroid gland. T3 is transported in the blood by a carrier protein called Thyroid Binding Globulin (TBG). The majority of your T3 thyroid hormone is bound and being transported by TBG. T3 is the hormone that packs the punch, and when unbound from TBG, directly affects the DNA of the cell. The only way T3 affects the cell is by being unbound from TBG. This measurement can be helpful because it helps determine both production of T3 from your thyroid gland and the amount that is being converted in the blood from T4.

Standard Range: 80 - 200 ng/dL

Optimal Range: >130 ng/dL

Free T3: This is still T3, but the unbound, or "free" portion of it. Remember, T3 is only effective when it is unbound from its carrier protein, TBG.

Standard Range: 2.3 - 4.2 pg/mL

Optimal Range: >3.0 pg/mL

Total T4: Total T4 is not always viewed as an important test in diagnosing hypothyroidism, but we disagree. Total T4 also reflects the production power of the thyroid because T4 is still the main hormone product produced by the thyroid gland. It can also imply if the patient has optimal nutrition. If T4 is on the high end, it can also indicate poor conversion of T4 into active T3 or the possible diagnosis of Thyroid Hormone Resistance (THR). THR is a condition where there is plenty of thyroid hormone being produced and available in the blood, but the target cells of the body are "resistant" to its positive stimulatory effects, leading to hypothyroidism (low thyroid).

Standard Range: 4.5 - 12.5 ug/dL

Optimal Range: >8.0 ug/dL

Free T4: This is the unbound version of T4, which can be even more accurate in helping to understand thyroid function.

Standard Range: 0.8 - 1.8 ng/dL

Optimal Range: >1.3 ng/dL

Reverse T3: This an often overlooked thyroid hormone by most conventional doctors. Reverse T3 is an *inactive* mirror image of regular active T3. Stress, high levels of cortisol, and very low caloric intake during extreme dieting will increase Reverse T3. The result of high levels of Reverse T3 lowers the metabolic rate by blocking the ability of regular active T3 to stimulate the cells of the body.

Standard Range: 8 – 25 ng/dL

Optimal Range: <15.0 ng/dL

Anti-TPO: During an autoimmune reaction (Hashimoto's) or inflammatory reaction (thyroiditis, postpartum thyroiditis) within the thyroid gland, the immune system will react to an enzyme called Thyroid Peroxidase (TPO). TPO is responsible for helping to complete the reaction of adding iodine to the amino acid tyrosine and therefore producing thyroid hormone, i.e. T4 or T3. When this value is elevated, it is demonstrating an autoimmune reaction in the body from some other source. It is important to note that the Anti-TPO value can be negative, but an inflammatory reaction could still be taking place within the thyroid gland.

Standard Range: <35 IU/mL

Optimal Range: <35 IU/mL

Anti-TG: Just like the Anti-TPO value, Anti-Thyroglobulin (Anti-TG) antibodies can reveal an autoimmune reaction that is occurring within the thyroid gland. Thyroglobulin is a necessary thyroid protein in the formation of thyroid hormone. During an immune reaction, the body produces antibodies against thyroglobulin called Anti-TG. Another important point about the Anti-TG value is that it is related to thyroid cancer. Fifteen to 30 percent of patients with a very elevated Anti-TG have thyroid cancer. If you have an elevated Anti-TG value, it would be wise to have a thyroid ultrasound to screen for the potential of thyroid cancer.

Standard Range: <4.0 IU/mL

Optimal Range: <4.0 IU/mL

Now that you have some understanding of the lab analysis and have seen the "optimal" ranges for these hormones, it is important to understand that your individual lab values still do not reveal everything. These values are suggesting an idea, a hypothesis, about what may be going on with your body and the thyroid gland itself. All lab values need to be interpreted not just by the raw value and the associated range, but within the overall clinical context of what is happening with the patient. This includes a strong consideration to the Resting Metabolic Rate (RMR) and Reflex Testing.

Step 5: Resting Metabolic Rate (RMR) & Reflex Testing

What if we told you that you could accurately and scientifically measure your metabolism, and this personal and unique measurement is related to your thyroid function? Sounds interesting, right? What if we also told you that this scientific measurement was more accurate than simply looking at thyroid blood tests? Now you may be even more interested. What if we told you that you could finally receive an accurate diagnosis about your suspected thyroid problems and then get the medical attention you know you've needed?

The answer is metabolic rate testing.

For decades, the use of metabolic rate testing has helped thyroid experts and physicians get a proper diagnosis for and monitor thyroid conditions. Once the easier (and less time consuming) blood analysis was discovered in the 1970s, the use of metabolic rate testing went out of fashion. There was a universal shift in all branches of medicine towards blood analysis as the main way to diagnosis and practice medicine. The practice of medicine was getting quicker and easier, but not necessarily more accurate in every situation.

Metabolic rate testing measures how fast the body consumes oxygen and this in turn helps you to understand how fast your metabolic rate is moving. Because your thyroid is the "master of metabolism," then this provides a very good idea about your thyroid's ability to produce thyroid hormone and regulate your metabolism.

ReeVue® Indirect Calorimetry

One of the best FDA approved metabolic rate testing devices available is the ReeVue® Indirect Calorimetry Measurement device. Let's get just a little technical and explain why metabolic rate testing works and how it will help you.

Metabolic rate testing measures the oxygen that your body consumes, and there is a direct correlation between it and the calories you burn. If you consume one millimeter of oxygen, you burn exactly 4.813 calories. Once this simple device measures how much oxygen your body consumes, you can multiply by 4.813

and this provides an accurate measurement of calorie consumption. This method is called indirect calorimetry. In the precise clinical setting with the ThyroZone system, the ReeVue® can be used to measure Basal Metabolic Rate (BMR) or the absolute lowest (basal) level of metabolic rate the body is producing. If the basal metabolic rate is abnormally low, then this assists in the diagnosis of hypothyroidism (low thyroid). If abnormally high, then hyperthyroidism (high thyroid) is considered.

The ThyroZone system uses a rational approach to the diagnosis and treatment of thyroid disorders by looking at the whole picture for a patient. Measuring metabolic rate is a large part of this. It takes a little more time, but you are worth it.

The ReeVue® test is used mostly for diagnostic purposes, but occasionally will be used for monitoring your metabolism while on your thyroid medication. It is initially used for diagnosis because it is highly accurate and helps to establish a baseline in a controlled clinical setting. Once you have your diagnosis and are in the process of improving your metabolism and thyroid gland with the ThyroZone system, monitoring can also be done with the ThyroFlex® instrument, explained below.

Having your metabolism checked with the ReeVue® is very simple. But there are a few things that are necessary to do to prepare for the test. Be sure to avoid food, caffeine, exercise, and all medications and herbal and nutritional supplements at least four hours before the test. Also:

Relax: ReeVue® measures your resting metabolic rate. It is important that you be able to reach a resting state during your test. At the time of the test, the lights are lowered, you are kept comfortable while lying covered with blankets, and soft music will be playing for about five to 10 minutes before the actual test begins and then throughout the duration of the test. This is all in an attempt to keep you as relaxed as possible.

Get 'Hooked Up': Lying relaxed and comfortable, you will have a nose clip placed on your nose and you will be given a disposable mouthpiece to breathe through. This mouthpiece is connected to the ReeVue® by a hose that measures how much oxygen you are breathing. It is very important that you breathe only through the mouthpiece so this measurement will be correct. Both the mouthpiece and the tubing are sterile items that will be used only for you.

Breathe: Just lay comfortably and breathe. The ReeVue® will indicate when it has calculated your RMR. This takes anywhere from five to 10 minutes. The more relaxed and even your breathing, the quicker it will be able to determine your RMR.

In a total of about 20 minutes, you will know precisely how many calories your body is burning, the speed of your personal metabolism, and your doctor will know how to properly diagnose and treat your possible thyroid condition.

Your RMR results will be printed and displayed on a range of either being "slow" or "fast". The *optimal* range is plus or minus (+/-) 5% of the predictive zero baseline. The *normal* range is at least plus or minus (+/-) 10%. If the RMR results show less than 10% this would be indicative of a slow metabolism and therefore hypothyroidism (low thyroid). If the results are greater than 10%, this would be indicative of a fast metabolism and therefore hyperthyroidism (high thyroid). These results will always be interpreted within the full context of your entire clinical picture.

Thyroflex®

One of the oldest and most accurate physical exams for diagnosing thyroid conditions is a deep tendon reflex test called Woltman's Sign. You are likely familiar with the idea behind this basic test. Your doctor uses a reflex hammer and hits you on your knee or on your elbow which helps to determine the function of your musculoskeletal and nervous systems, and as you will see, determines your metabolic speed and thyroid function.

About a hundred years ago, physicians observed that the condition of either hypothyroidism (low thyroid) or hyperthyroidism (high thyroid) directly affected the reflexes of the body. In hypothyroidism, the reflexes are slow. In hyperthyroidism, the reflexes are fast. In the past, doctors would have to use the basic reflex hammer tool and with merely a keen eye, determine if the reflex speed was too slow or too fast. It is an acquired skill but even the most skilled physician can have difficulty in measuring the exact speed of the reflex.

The Thyroflex® has helped to make the use of reflex speed assessment for thyroid disorders even more accurate, helping you to optimize your thyroid medication dose and your personal metabolism.

The ThyroFlex® was designed by Konrad Kail, P.A., N.D., and Daryl Turner, Ph.D. after years of research. It was produced for medical use by 2007 and has been helping thousands of patients all over the world ever since. Understanding that reflex speed has been used in thyroid disease diagnosis and treatment, they brought this time-tested medical tool into the 21st century with accurate and reproducible computer-aided technology. The ThyroFlex® accurately examines the brachioradialis reflex speed, a reflex found near your elbow that makes your wrist move up and down.

Because your reflexes are associated with your metabolism, they are also associated with your thyroid function, the master of metabolism. The ThyroFlex® also determines your Resting Metabolic Rate (RMR) which is the amount of calories your body is burning at rest. This is the same thing the ReeVue® machine does, except it is using a calculation based off of your reflex speed.

The optimal range for your ThyroFlex® test results is 50 to 100 milliseconds. Faster than 50 milliseconds may indicate hyper-thyroidism (high thyroid) or an excessive amount of thyroid hormone medication. Between 100 to 135 milliseconds implies a possible nutritional deficiency such as iodine, without necessarily being a complete diagnosis of hypothyroidism (low thyroid). However, other clinical signs and symptoms may still strongly point to hypothyroidism. Once the reflex speed is above 136 milliseconds, hypothyroidism and a lowered metabolic rate is highly likely. Just as with the RMR, these results will be interpreted within the full context of your entire clinical picture.

Step 6: Other Clinical Diagnostic Tools

Thyroid Ultrasound

A thyroid ultrasound is a very simple and painless diagnostic procedure using ultrasonography. It helps to determine the exact size of the thyroid gland and determine if goiter (enlargement of the thyroid gland) is present. Thyroid ultrasound also helps to determine if there are fluid filled nodules (cysts) or solid nodules. Solid nodules greater than about one to one and a half centimeters in diameter usually need a biopsy to rule out thyroid cancer. Thyroid nodules are very common and do not necessarily indicate a major problem, but can be indicative of a nutritional deficiency or a general thyroid dysfunction such as hypothyroidism (low thyroid).

You will need a thyroid ultrasound if:

- You have the suspicion of goiter or nodules or other masses based on clinical physical exam.
- You have an enlarged thyroid based on clinical physical exam and it is NOT painful (this is usually indicative of

an autoimmune condition specifically known as Hashimoto's thyroiditis).

- You have an enlarged thyroid based on clinical physical exam and it IS painful (this is still considered thyroiditis, or inflammation of the thyroid gland, but it may or may not be from an underlying autoimmune condition).
- You have enlarged lymph nodes under your chin (submandibular) and/or along your neck (not from an acute infection), along with a possible enlarged thyroid (goiter) or difficulty swallowing or an enlarged tongue (usually is accompanied with pain).
- Your thyroid blood work demonstrates an elevated anti-TG value which may be associated with thyroid cancer.
- Your thyroid blood work demonstrates an elevated anti-TPO and/or an elevated anti-TG which indicates Hashimoto's thyroiditis.
- You have a history of thyroid cancer but did not have your thyroid gland completely removed.
- You have a history of having a thyroid ultrasound that found anything abnormal including thyroid nodules, thyroid cysts, or goiter.

Thyroid Biopsy

Depending on the results of your physical exam, or from a possible thyroid ultrasound, you may need to have a tissue sample removed from your thyroid gland in a very simple procedure using Fine Needle Aspiration (FNA).

You will need a thyroid biopsy if:

Any one nodule is from 1 to 1.5 cm or greater in diameter.

A pattern of microcalcifications is found within the thyroid gland on ultrasound (microcalcifications are deposits of calcium of unknown origin but are strongly correlated with cancerous tumors with a predictive value of up to 95 percent). In other words, if you have microcalcifications found on your thyroid ultrasound, the likelihood of thyroid cancer is very high and you will need to have this examined further.

Thyroid Thermography

Thermography is a medical imaging tool that uses digital infrared imaging, that measures heat signatures in tissues such as the thyroid gland. Thermography is based on the principle that metabolic activity and blood circulation in precancerous tissue and the area surrounding a developing cancer is usually higher than normal tissue. Cancerous tumors are metabolically greedy, and increase circulation to their cells by increasing blood supply to existing blood vessels, opening dormant vessels, and creating new ones in a process known as neoangiogenesis. There is a copious amount of medical research supporting the use of thermography as a diagnostic aid for decades.

The ThyroZone system promotes the use of thermography to determine the physiology (function) of the thyroid gland to determine hypothyroidism (low thyroid) and hyperthyroidism (high thyroid) because temperature signatures are generally *lower* in hypothyroidism and *higher* in hyperthyroidism. Thermography will also help to identify inflammatory states such as Hashimoto's thyroiditis or Grave's disease, and even structural changes such as goiter (enlarged thyroid), thyroid nodules, and potential cancerous thyroid tumors. In the case of any structural changes, it is encouraged to have a thyroid ultrasound for supportive imaging information, and additional medical referrals.

The process of having a thyroid thermograph test is extremely simple. Using a high-tech camera, the technician takes several views of the thyroid gland. There is no pain or radiation exposure from this process. It's simply a picture. The data is then stored and sent to a Board Certified Radiologist who interprets the results and sends a report to your doctor for review. The Thyro-Zone system uses thyroid thermography as an additional tool to create diagnosis and track your progressive improvement.

Electrocardiogram (ECG)

An electrocardiogram (ECG) is a simple test measuring the electric conduction of the heart muscle. Thyroid hormone is extremely important for a healthy heart and there are several non-specific changes in your ECG that could occur in either hypothyroidism (low thyroid) or hyperthyroidism (high thyroid). The ThyroZone system uses your ECG results to establish a diagnosis of low thyroid and low metabolism. Your cardiac safety with thyroid hormone medication may also be assessed through the ECG result. However, the main use of the ECG is for close monitoring while you're on thyroid hormone medication. Because most patients benefiting from the ThyroZone system will be on doses of thyroid hormone medication that suppresses the Thyroid Stimulating Hormone (TSH) lab value to near zero, it is important to monitor heart function. When the TSH is very low, hyperthyroidism (high thyroid) and elevated metabolism are considered clinically and the ECG is a tool used to demonstrate that your optimal thyroid hormone dose is safe for your heart. Remember that the TSH blood test value is extremely poor at determining what is happening with your body and how you feel.

The main cardiac issue that can be easily determined by an ECG is atrial fibrillation or "a-fib." This is when the smaller chambers of the heart (called the atria) beat too rapidly and not in coordination with the rest of the heart, and blood can pool and clot. If atrial fibrillation is found, then a referral to a cardiologist would be necessary to have more advanced testing.

Be sure to refer to Chapter 7 on monitoring your progress for more information on what to look out for with your ECG findings.

Step 7: Common Diet Factors in Thyroid Disease

Your personal daily diet affects everything about your health. Your thyroid gland health is directly correlated to the quality of your diet.

In some cases, people react to food in ways that will induce thyroid disease. If you can control your diet, you can often control your thyroid condition, and certainly improve how you feel. Let's explore some of the specific aspects of food that can lead to thyroid disease.

Lectins: One Autoimmune Culprit

Lectins are small proteins that bind carbohydrate molecules. Lectins are found in every type of food to some degree, but high levels are found in all grains (particularly wheat), legumes (like peanuts), dairy, and plants in the nightshade family, such as potatoes and peppers. Lectins have the ability to bind to molecules within the cell membrane of any body cell, including your thyroid cells, and lead to an autoimmune reaction. Lectins are known as "anti-nutrients" or chemical strategies to protect them from predators, especially when they are still unripe. Some of the other chemical protection strategies are inhibitors of your own saliva production, like trypsin and α-amylase inhibitor. Other chemical anti-nutrients include phytic acid and nitrates. While they are designed to protect the plant, anti-nutrients lead to your poor health.

How Lectins Affect the Thyroid Gland

Lectins act like keys in the way they bind to the thyroid's TSH receptors. We call this a "Long-Acting Thyroid Stimulator"

(LATS). When there is an over-abundance of lectins present in the bloodstream it can lead to over-stimulation of the thyroid gland that creates an autoimmune reaction, which then leads to two different possible negative reactions.

One, LATS can lead to the autoimmune condition known as Grave's disease, which leads to overproduction of thyroid hormones, or hyperthyroidism (high thyroid).

Two, LATS will create the autoimmune condition known as Hashimoto's thyroiditis and, instead of stimulating the TSH receptor, it *blocks* the TSH receptor. This lowers production of thyroid hormones and leads to hypothyroidism (low thyroid).

What Can You Do About Lectins in Your Food?

First, avoid them. Reducing grain-based carbohydrates is, in general, a good idea for your thyroid and your waistline. Another way to deal with lectins is to neutralize them in the way food is prepared. One method to reduce lectin content is to sprout grains and beans that you may eat. Soaking grains and beans helps to eliminate anti-nutrients because it mimics the natural sprouting or germination process. Germination in the wild leads to eliminating anti-nutrients that are largely found in the outer skin coating. Sprouting as a food preparation process has been done for thousands of years and is completely consistent with the Traditional Ancestral Diet.

Gluten: Another Autoimmune Culprit

Gluten is the main protein found in wheat, barley, and rye. There is mounting evidence that the gluten protein in wheat is associated with autoimmune thyroid disease including Hashimoto's thyroiditis (low thyroid) and Grave's disease (high thyroid). People with definitive celiac disease have a 25 percent chance of having some type of thyroid condition. This connection has been understood for years but little is ever done at the clinical level, such as automatic testing for gluten intolerance and diet counseling on how to avoid gluten. But with the ThyroZone system, we explore this possibility.

By now, most people have heard of gluten-free food products. More and more people understand that gluten and wheat products cause them gastrointestinal discomfort and a multitude of other symptoms. Some people have very obvious reactions to gluten, but many people who have serious health issues related to gluten never really make the connection. Many of the symptoms related to gluten have nothing to do with the gastrointestinal tract. Let's explore some of the symptoms of gluten intolerance now.

Symptoms of Gluten Intolerance

Weight gain

Fatigue

Insomnia

Craving baked goods and high sugar foods

Intestinal bloating or gas after eating

IBS: Irritable Bowel Syndrome

Acid reflux and indigestion

Constipation and/or diarrhea

Frequent nausea and/or vomiting

Headaches and sinus congestion

Migraine headaches

Vertigo

Poor memory

Brain fog

Depression and anxiety

Numbness and tingling

Irritability and mood swings

Muscle aches and joint pain

Psoriasis

Eczema

Dermatitis

Skin rashes and itching

Yeast infections

Restless Leg Syndrome

Diagnosed of ADD (Attention Deficit Disorder)

Diagnosed with Chronic Fatigue Syndrome

Diagnosed with Fibromyalgia

Diagnosed with Multiple Sclerosis or Parkinson's

Diagnosed with any autoimmune condition

Diagnosed with endometriosis

Leaky Gut Syndrome

Now that we understand that both lectins and gluten negatively affect the immune system and thyroid health, let's explore the results of what they do to the digestive system. One of the eventual consequences is something called Leaky Gut Syndrome. When the proteins between cells within your digestive track begin to break down including the digestive cells themselves, larger proteins and other components of the digestive tract get into the general circulation. Normally these proteins would not get into the general circulation, because the digestive tract would assimilate and detoxify them. Once the larger proteins are through the protective layer of the digestive tract, this leads to immune reactions to the perceived "invaders," malabsorption of important nutrients, and excess toxicity. Certain blood tests can show evidence of Leaky Gut Syndrome, which would include measuring antibody (immune soldier) reactions against the proteins that bind digestive tract cells together.

Leaky Gut Symptoms and Signs

Increased food sensitivities

Autoimmune diseases such as Hashimoto's or Grave's disease

Skin conditions such as dermatitis and rashes

Joint pain and arthritis

Inflammatory bowel disease

Malabsorption syndrome

Mental and emotional disturbances

Common Causes of Leaky Gut Syndrome

Medications such as NSAIDS

Bacterial or viral infections

Genetic susceptibility

Environmental toxins such as pesticides

Overconsumption of grains and wheat

Proper Testing for Gluten Intolerance

Celiac disease is an intense and specific immune reaction to eating gluten, a protein found in wheat, barley, and rye. The reactions to gluten are very extreme and generally very obvious after eating it, including gas, bloating, cramping, and severe diarrhea that is pale and foul smelling. Celiac disease leads to serious malabsorption of nutrients and increases the future risk of cancers in the digestive tract. Diagnosis often involves a basic blood test, an endoscopy (scope in the intestines) and a possible biopsy tissue sample of the intestines. Many people react to gluten and wheat proteins but do not have the more serious condition of celiac disease. This is an important distinction.

As mentioned before, gluten intolerance can still be present in someone even if they do not have the diagnosis of celiac disease. In fact, many people have a reaction to gluten *and* the non-gluten wheat proteins found in wheat. Or, they react to the non-gluten wheat proteins but not the gluten. It is important to make the distinction. Many people actually react to non-gluten wheat proteins, but are ok with gluten. For those that react to both, then gluten-free breads, as an example, would still be a problem because it still contains wheat proteins.

Make sure the testing you chose for gluten intolerance has the following components:

Celiac panel

Gliadin and glutenin (gluten proteins)

Non-gluten wheat proteins

Step 8: Common Thyroid Environmental Toxins and Endocrine Disruptors

Environmental toxins are everywhere. Their negative effects are far-reaching and your endocrine system and thyroid gland are not immune. In fact, the endocrine system is one of the main body systems affected by environmental toxins. These toxins have been given the special designation of endocrine disruptors.

Here is a specific list of environmental toxins known to be associated with causing autoimmune thyroid disease:

PCBs: Found in coolants and lubricants

Organochlorine pesticides: Used as a pesticide on crops

PBDEs: Found in flame retardants

BPA: Used in plastic bottles

Perchlorate and thiocyanate: Rocket fuel, fertilizer, smoking

Triclosan: Antibacterial in soaps

Isoflavones: Soy products

What to do next is fairly obvious. Simply avoid these things as much as possible. There are so many alternatives available now making it is fairly easy. Eat organic, avoid plastics in contact with your food and water, don't smoke, use regular soap and avoid soy food products other than fermented soy.

Step 9: Comprehensive Diagnosis: Bringing it Together

Now that you and your doctor have followed through with all of the diagnostic elements of the ThyroZone system, you need to ask some questions to know what to do next:

1. Are the clinical symptoms heavily weighted to thyroid disease?
2. Did the results of the hypothyroid questionnaire, the Zulewski's Hypothyroid Clinical Score, and the Wayne's Hyperthyroid Index indicate a possible dysfunction?
3. Do you also have the typically associated diseases such as hypertension (high blood pressure) or insulin resistance and diabetes?
4. What were the results of your ThyroFlex® score? Was it slow, indicating hypothyroidism (low thyroid) or was it fast, indicating hyperthyroidism (high thyroid)?
5. What were the results of your RMR using the ReeVue® machine? Was if slow or fast?
6. What were the results of your ECG? Did it show atrial fibrillation (a-fib)?
7. Did you get all of the suggested thyroid labs?
8. Did your results fall into the optimal ranges, particularly your TSH and your Free T3?
9. Did you have elevated antibodies such as anti-TPO or anti-TG?

10. Was it found on clinical exam that you have an enlarged thyroid gland?
11. If it was necessary, what were the results of your thyroid ultrasound? Did it show an enlarged thyroid gland or possible enlarged nodules? Did the thyroid ultrasound results list a "heterogenous" appearance to the thyroid gland tissue, indicating Hashimoto's?
12. Did you need a biopsy of any nodules greater than 1 to 1.5 cm? What were the results?
13. What were the results of your thyroid thermograph? Did it show cold or hot areas in and around your thyroid gland?
14. Was it found that you have a gluten and/or wheat sensitivity? Do you consume a lot of unfermented soy products?
15. Are you avoiding as many endocrine disruptor chemicals as possible? Are you considering safer, more natural alternative products when you can?

This chapter covered a thorough analysis of your thyroid gland health and your metabolic health. With this information, you will know how to properly treat the issue and monitor your progress. Maybe you are starting to see the big picture about your thyroid, one way or another. But for as thorough as all of this is, it does not replace the advice and guidance of a healthcare professional, although it does arm you with more insight than some of the most seasoned doctors. Most important is that it helps you to start helping yourself.

Individualized Thyroid Treatment

Often patients believe they have a thyroid condition, particularly hypothyroidism (low thyroid), but this may or may not be true. The ThyroZone system is designed to help you understand why you feel they way you do. Our practice succeeds where other medical models fail because the ThyroZone system provides a comprehensive clinical framework characterized by an open-minded assessment of your condition, a review of potential environmental and other disease causing factors, an accurate clinical diagnosis and customized treatment and monitoring.

Support the Thyroid First, Even in Borderline Cases

This medical approach is to your advantage because the multiple angles used to heal the thyroid will ultimately heal the entire body. If your diagnosis is "borderline," the first step in treatment is to support the thyroid gland and your metabolism, before deciding to prescribe thyroid hormone medication.

By starting with supporting the thyroid and its optimal function, we achieve several things:

1. With a less invasive approach to treating the thyroid, we allow the gland to support itself and the body.

2. We support the metabolism, which is the underlying reason for the symptoms (remember that thyroid symptoms, whether low or high, are from either a low or high metabolic rate).

3. We treat the underlying cause of the perceived hypothyroidism (low thyroid), such as gluten intolerance, toxicity, nutritional deficiencies, mitochondrial dysfunction, and other hormonal deficiencies such as menopausal estrogen deficiency, or adrenal dysfunction.

4. We can make a clinical diagnosis of thyroid hormone deficiency if the patient is not improving significantly within a reasonable amount of time. (If after 8 to 12 weeks of supporting the thyroid in this fashion, there is no marked improvement, then a deeper problem is likely present and it is reasonable to take the therapy to the next step.)

Through this comprehensive symptom management process, we successfully achieve several goals: strengthen the body, maximize its potential to use thyroid hormone, and inevitably, improve treatment outcomes. In other words, this whole conservative approach of healing the thyroid is a win-win strategy.

From a clinical standpoint, there is a logical sequence in the optimal treatment of thyroid and metabolic disorders, whether you are taking thyroid hormone medication or not. So, consider them carefully, and start by asking: How would you know if this is where you should start, instead of seeking to be on thyroid medication right away?

The decision to medicate is based on several factors.

1. The severity of your symptoms based on results from the Zulewski's Clinical Score for hypothyroidism (low thyroid) or Wayne's Hyperthyroid Index for hyperthyroidism (high thyroid) and, other clinical signs and symptoms. Your physician should discuss this with you if you are borderline, or perhaps just under the scale.

2. The results of your ThyroFlex® test. This test provides a suboptimal range prior to the diagnosis of hypothyroidism (low thyroid) where it would be wise to support the thyroid before considering thyroid hormone medication.

3. The results of your Resting Metabolic Rate (RMR) test with the ReeVue®. In the same respect as the ThyroFlex®, consider support with an RMR result that is barely out of the optimal range.

4. Thyroid lab results that are not significantly suboptimal, even with the tighter ranges suggested in the ThyroZone system.

If you first considered your thyroid condition as borderline, and you and your physician have sufficiently exhausted these options, then move onto consider thyroid hormone medication. If you have a significant initial presentation of hypothyroidism (low thyroid), then you would be prescribed thyroid hormone medication *but* you would *still* need to consider the other steps in this chapter to get the best results. If you have a significant presentation of hyperthyroidism (high thyroid), then these symptoms necessitate immediate medical intervention; but, again, the other steps would still need to be considered.

The Thyroid Diet

In general, the best diet for your body, and your thyroid, is the Traditional Ancestral Diet. It focuses on high fat, moderate protein, and moderately low carbohydrates, properly prepared through soaking and fermentation. In our practice, and throughout *The Hormone Zone* book, both Dr. Bosch and Dr. Robinson have discussed and promoted the Paleo Diet with our patients for years. We still believe that this diet is good because of its perspective of viewing nutrition through the lens of how our ancestors ate. There are over 40 cultures that still live and eat "traditionally" (as humans have eaten for thousands of years) that we observe and study. These cultures were also observed and studied by the renowned dentist and scientist Weston A. Price and his wife nearly 100 years ago. The conclusions of Price, brilliantly laid out in his seminal work *Nutrition and Physical Degeneration*, and the observations and conclusions of current anthropologists, reveal that there are distinct differences between the Paleo Diet and the Traditional Ancestral Diet. We believe these differences to be distinct and medically imperative towards optimal health and longevity.

You can review the differences between the Traditional Ancestral Diet (aka The Weston A. Price Foundation Diet) and the Paleo Diet on the Weston A. Price Foundation website. (Please refer to the Resources section of this book for specific website information.) For now, one of the key differences is based on the recommendation of fats. The Paleo Diet recommends animal meats that are lean, with little fat. The Traditional Ancestral Diet recommends animal meats with their fat intact, along with the coveted high-fat organ meats.

Of the people in traditional cultures who've been the focus of diet studies, there were none that thrived on low fat diets. As a matter of fact, in the ancestral diet, fat is king. Fat is the vehicle that traditional peoples use to flourish with optimal health. The same can be for you, for your health, and certainly for your thyroid.

How to Eat a Traditional Ancestral Diet

This is one of the healthiest ways to eat. Humans have been eating this diet for thousands of years. Weston A. Price traveled the world studying various peoples who had a traditional ancestral diet. Here is an overview (paraphrased from information on his website) of what his vast travels and keen observations have shown:

1. The diets of healthy primitive and non-industrialized peoples contain no refined or denatured foods.
2. All traditional cultures consume animal protein and fat from fish and other seafood; water and land fowl; land animals; eggs; milk and milk products; reptiles; and insects.
3. Primitive diets contain at least four times the calcium and other minerals, and *ten* times the fat soluble vitamins, from animal fats (vitamin A, D3, E, and K2) as the average American diet.
4. In all traditional cultures, some animal products are eaten raw.
5. Primitive and traditional diets have a high food-enzyme content from raw dairy products raw meat and fish; raw honey; tropical fruits; cold-pressed oils; wine and unpasteurized beer; and naturally preserved, lacto-fermented vegetables, fruits, beverages, meats and condiments.
6. Seeds, grains and nuts are soaked, sprouted, fermented or

naturally leavened in order to neutralize naturally occurring anti-nutrients in these foods, such as phytic acid, enzyme inhibitors, tannins and complex carbohydrates.

7. Total fat content of traditional diets varies from 30 to 80 percent but only about 4 percent of calories come from polyunsaturated oils that naturally occur in grains, pulses, edible seeds, nuts, fish, animal fats and vegetables. The balance of fat calories is in the form of saturated and monounsaturated fatty acids.

8. Traditional diets contain nearly equal amounts of omega-6 and omega-3 essential fatty acids.

9. All primitive diets contain some salt.

10. Traditional cultures consume animal bones, usually in the form of gelatin-rich bone broths.

11. Traditional cultures make provisions for the health of future generations by providing special nutrient-rich foods for parents-to-be, pregnant women and growing children; by proper spacing of children; and by teaching the principles of right diet to the young.

Goitrogens

A goitrogen is a substance that has a tendency to either block the production of thyroid hormone or alter the action of thyroid hormone on cells. Goitrogenic foods possess the potential to lower thyroid function. But this idea is overstated and, in general, there is little clinical evidence to support this claim. Eating these foods, even raw, will not readily cause a goiter or low thyroid condition.

However, where we have seen this to be an issue is with *raw* vegetable juice when it's consumed in large amounts. We are seeing a trend of raw juice bars that feature kale. Because juice is so highly concentrated, and because some people are now eating these types of drinks so frequently, it is then possible to have a goitrogenic, or thyroid lowering, effect. There is certainly a potential problem with consuming excessive raw kale juice because of the high oxalate content that can potentially contribute to kidney stone formation.

Most goitrogenic foods will be neutralized if they are cooked. The exception to this is soy, canola oil, and rapeseed. Most of the soy that is consumed is highly processed, often in the form of Genetically Modified Organism (GMO) soybean oil, a highly goitrogenic food that interferes with thyroid function and increases autoimmunity. Canola oil, derived from rapeseed, is used as an effective non-chemical insecticide and is not fit for human consumption. It increases the omega-6 to omega-3 ratio to beyond the one-to-one ideal and is highly sensitive to oxidation when heated.

Eating a Traditional Ancestral Diet will take care of any potential issues or concerns over goitrogenic foods. Remember that the majority of the foods listed here are absolutely fine to eat, but are listed for clarity. Just avoid consuming unfermented soy, canola oil and rapeseed unless prepared in a fermented state or cooked in some way, thereby neutralizing the anti-nutrients and lectins.

List of Typical Goitrogen Foods

Bamboo shoots
Bok Choy
Genus *Brassica* vegtables (in the mustard family)
Broccoli
Broccolini
Brussels sprouts

Cabbage

Canola oil (rapeseed)

Cassava

Cauliflower

Choy sum

Collard greens

Horseradish

Kale

Kohlrabi

Millet

Mizuna

Mustard greens

Peaches

Peanuts

Pears

Pine nuts

Radishes

Rapeseed

Rapini

Rutabagas

Soy (unfermented)

Spinach

Strawberries

Sweet potato

Tatsoi

Turnips

A Word About Soy and the Thyroid

For the sake of your thyroid gland health you should avoid *unfermented* soy products, such as tofu, raw edamame, Texturized Vegetable Protein (TVP, soy 'meat' or soy protein isolate), soybean oil, soymilk, soy cheese, soy ice cream, soy yogurt, soy protein added to foods or soy protein powders, and soy infant formula. Many soy products are hidden in packaged foods, so be sure to read labels.

The two main soy isoflavones, genistein and daidzein, both inhibit thyroid peroxidase, the enzyme involved in thyroid hormone synthesis. In the presence of these isoflavones, you will not produce the thyroid hormones T4 and T3. These are usually produced from tyrosine and iodine. Instead, your body will produce a useless mixture of soy isoflavones, iodine, and tyrosine. It's both interesting and frightening that researchers use thyroid hormone medication with a combination of soy isoflavones in experimental lab rats to induce thyroid tumors.

Fermented soy is a very different product altogether, but is not the type of soy that is most often eaten in the United States. Japan is very well known for their consumption of *fermented* soy and its related health benefits. The fermentation process neutralizes the soy isoflavones and other anti-nutrients found in soy, helping your thyroid and your health. Examples are the fermented soybean cake, tempeh; miso, a fermented soybean paste used in soups; natto, a pungent, strong fermented sticky soybean; and soy sauce, which is fermented soybean when traditionally made. These types of soy are recommended and are *not* goitrogenic. Notice that fermented soy is consistent with the Traditional Ancestral Diet we've recommended in this chapter.

Common Goitrogenic Medications

The medications below are listed because they are common and have more of an impact to developing a goiter (enlarged thyroid) than the goitrogenic foods. There is really no comparison between these goitrogenic medications and foods in their ability to cause goiter and thyroid dysfunction. Be sure to discuss your thyroid health with your doctor if you have been prescribed these medications:

- Anti-thyroid medications for treating hyperthyroidism such as Tapazole® (methimazole) and propylthiouracil.
- The antibiotics called sulfonamides.
- The anti-arrhythmic heart medication called Cardarone® (amiodarone).
- The bipolar medication lithium.
- The ulcerative colitis medication Salofalk®.
- The tuberculosis medications ethionamide and amino-salicylate sodium.

Lectins and Gluten: The Autoimmune Culprits in Hashimoto's Thyroiditis and Grave's Disease

We discussed gluten and lectins in Chapter 5. Also recall that Hashimoto's thyroiditis is the autoimmune disease that leads to hypothyroidism (low thyroid) and Grave's disease is the autoimmune disease leading to hyperthyroidism (high thyroid). Remember, the term "autoimmune" refers to the process where your own immune system becomes triggered and produces antibodies, a type of immune soldier, to attack various tissues within your own (auto or self) body, including your thyroid gland.

So what can you do about these lectins? What's the treatment? You already know the answer—avoid them! By largely following the Traditional Ancestral Diet, you'll drastically reduce your intake of lectins.

Now let's see how gluten affects your thyroid gland.

Gluten

If you determined by now that you have gluten intolerance, and if you have elevated thyroid antibodies such as Anti-TPO or Anti-TG, then what can you do? You guessed it, avoid gluten and wheat. It is that simple, but yet so profound for how you will feel. You will actually be working on the cause of your thyroid disorder instead of just band-aiding the problem.

We have seen profound results in patients with Hashimoto's thyroiditis and Grave's disease who simply avoided gluten and wheat. Another important point here to make is that by following the Traditional Ancestral Diet described here, you largely avoid gluten and wheat. Here's a more specific list of foods that contain wheat:

- Wheat, including forms of wheat like bulgur, couscous, durum, farina, farro, kamut, matzoh, semolina, spelt, and triticale
- Barley, including brewer's yeast, malt, malt extract and flavoring, and malt vinegar
- Rye, including breads and cereals
- Hidden sources of gluten include: baby food, candy such as chocolate and licorice, soy sauce, gravies and marinades, tortillas, processed meats, malted milk shakes, salad dressing, soups, processed and packaged foods, mixed spice blends, ice creams, puddings, spreads and dips, and some medications and supplements.

Precise Nutritional and Botanical Tools

The ThyroZone system seeks to provide you with the best nutritional strategies for your thyroid health and your entire body. Nutritional and herbal tools are integral parts of this strategy. When correcting the metabolism with adequate thyroid hormone, the body needs additional nutritional support. Professional grade supplements achieve the best results.

They are the oil for the body's engine!

We believe there are many nutrients that are important for your body and your thyroid gland. There are volumes written on the long list of nutrients that can be beneficial, but listing them all, and therefore asking a patient to take them all, is simply not practical. We have done our best to provide the most important nutrients here. There may be others that will part of your personal nutritional plan for your thyroid health.

The Top Nutrients for Your Thyroid Gland

The place to start with is what we call "the basics."

The Basics

What you should be taking, whether for thyroid health or general health, are well-known and readily available but please note that all of them should be of "professional quality" in order to guarantee potency, quality and effectiveness.

The great thing about these basic components is they have far-reaching health implications beyond just your thyroid gland. You will cover many nutritional bases by including the nutrients listed here:

- Multivitamin and mineral complex: 1 daily
- Fish oil: 2000-3000 mg daily
- Vitamin D3: 5,000 to 10,000 IU daily
- Vitamin K2: 150 to 200 mcg daily
- Probiotic: Professional potency, 100 Billion CFUs, 1 daily

Going Beyond the Basics

There are six other supplements we consider to be important to your overall metabolic health. Again, look for high quality physician-grade when you purchase them.

Iodine

Iodine is the most important nutrient for the thyroid gland. Thyroid hormone is composed of the amino acid tyrosine surrounded by three or four iodine molecules. Without iodine, there is no thyroid hormone. However, iodine has far reaching benefits for your thyroid gland beyond making thyroid hormone.

In the book *The Hormone Zone*, an entire chapter is devoted to the wonders of this nutrient. Iodine is important for breast health, lowering the risk for breast cancer and treating fibrocystic breast disease. It enhances the immune system and has been shown to increase IQ in children who receive it in utero and as young children. It increases the metabolic rate, improves energy and lifts brain fog. It is very effective as a detoxifier of heavy metals such as lead and mercury and also detoxifies the effects of halides (halogen molecule compounds) such as fluoride (found in toothpaste and our water supply) and bromide (used as a dough conditioner in bread).

In cases of hypothyroidism (low thyroid), one of the most important reasons to give iodine to any patient who is on thyroid hormone medication is because it helps the thyroid hormone work more efficiently in the presence of adequate thyroid hormone. Suggested dose for hypothyroidism: 12.5 to 50 mg of potassium iodine/iodide, along with 200 mcg of selenium. Selenium should always be giving when taking iodine supplementation. For patients taking thyroid hormone medication, the usual dose is 12.5 mg daily. In hyperthyroidism (high thyroid) cases, higher doses are extremely effective at helping to lower thyroid hormone levels and normalize the thyroid gland. Suggested dosing for hyperthyroidism: 12.5 mg to 50 mg daily, or higher. The use of iodine therapy in hyperthyroidism should be used only under the direction of a physician.

Selenium

The thyroid gland has the highest selenium content per gram of tissue than any other organ because selenium works with iodine to produce thyroid hormone. In the autoimmune disease Hashimoto's (the one that results in low thyroid), and in pregnant women with elevated Anti-TPO antibodies, selenium supplementation decreases those antibody levels and improves the structure of the thyroid gland.

In the autoimmune disease, Graves' disease, that results in hyperthyroidism (high thyroid), selenium supplementation helps to normalize the thyroid gland more rapidly and improves the eye swelling that is common with the disease. Suggested dose: 200 mcg daily.

Zinc

Zinc is responsible for helping your body to convert inactive T4 thyroid hormone into the active T3 hormone. This mineral is also necessary for the T3 receptor of your cells to function properly. If the T3 receptor does not work properly, then even adequate levels of T3 thyroid hormone will be less useful and result in thyroid symptoms. Suggested dose: 30 to 90 mcg daily.

Magnesium

Magnesium is responsible for hundreds of chemical reactions in your body, yet it is one of the most common mineral deficiencies. Specifically for the thyroid, magnesium is responsible for converting the inactive T4 thyroid hormone into the active form of T3. This is extremely important because the metabolism of your body's cells is enhanced by T3, not inactive T4. Magnesium deficiency is also related to goiter, or an enlarged thyroid gland. Also, magnesium helps you to make more T4 in the thyroid gland.

There are several types of magnesium. For example, if you have constipation, then consider magnesium citrate, a version that helps to move the bowels. Otherwise, consider magnesium glycinate or magnesium taurate, both versions assist with calming the mind and inducing relaxation.

Without magnesium, many of the thyroid enzymes that make thyroid hormone simply could not function. In addition to the many benefits of magnesium for your thyroid gland, there is a long list of general benefits to your body including relieving such symptoms as muscle aches and pains, numbness and tingling, fatigue, constipation, and much more. Suggested Dose: 400 to 1200 mg nightly.

Vitamin A

This fat-soluble vitamin is extremely important for your overall health as well as the health of your thyroid gland. Vitamin A has been shown to lower TSH and increase T3 levels, both of which help to correct hypothyroidism (low thyroid). It can also decrease goiter (enlarged thyroid) and reduces the autoimmune response in Hashimoto's. Suggested Dose: 10,000 IU Daily of Retinol.

Vitamin D

One of the most important nutrients in your body, vitamin D actually operates like a hormone, stimulating the thyroid gland and its receptors. Its immune stimulation and regulatory functions are profound. For those with the autoimmune conditions Hashimoto's or Grave's disease, vitamin D is extremely important. Low levels of vitamin D are also associated with thyroid cancer. Be sure to have your 25-hydroxy vitamin D levels checked and properly monitored before starting vitamin D supplementation. Suggested dose: 2,000 to 10,000 IU of vitamin D3 daily.

Botanical Tools

There are many herbs that have the ability to help with thyroid function and balance. The two that we have found have the most direct benefit are *Fucus vesiculosus* or bladderwrack, a form of seaweed, and *Melissa officinalis*, or lemon balm.

Fucus vesiculosus

Fucus is the genus name of a seaweed variety in use and consumed by humans for thousands of years. It is highly nutritious and is an excellent source of iodine, the key nutrient in thyroid hormone. Fucus vesiculosus, or commonly Bladderwrack, actually contains small amounts of the slightly active thyroid hormone T2, as well as the components to assist in synthesizing active T3. In large enough quantities, it has potent metabolism stimulating effects, and is used for hypothyroid (low thyroid) patients. Suggested dose: 1 to 10 grams; start slowly and increase by one gram daily.

Melissa officinalis

This herb, also known as lemon balm, is used for patients with hyperthyroidism (high thyroid). It contains rosmarinic acid, a component that will bind with Thyroid Stimulating Hormone (TSH) and the TSH receptor, rendering them less effective and thereby lowering the hyperactivity of the thyroid gland. It also binds with Thyroid Stimulating Immunoglobins (TSI), the antibodies associated with hyperthyroidism and Grave's disease. It helps to calm the nervous system and the heart, as well as aid in digestion, which are all common symptoms in hyperthyroidism. There are no known side effects of this herb. It is important to take a professionally prepared tincture that is potent enough to provide the medicinal effect.

Suggested Dose: 2-2.5 mL of a 1:3 extract.

Detoxification and Your Thyroid

Due to the significant blood supply to the thyroid gland, it is highly vulnerable to toxins. Many thyroid conditions are induced by exposure to environmental toxins, so avoiding exposure and considering proper detoxification are the first steps to helping your thyroid gland.

Avoiding Common Thyroid Toxins

The first step in detoxifying your body and your thyroid from toxins is to avoid them in the first place. Here is a list of seven known everyday chemicals that disrupt thyroid function and what alternatives exist to replace them:

1. Bromide. Found in soft drinks—which should be avoided as a general rule for good health. Replace with carbonated water flavored with 100 percent fruit juice.
2. Fluoride. Found in drinking water and toothpaste. Drink only filtered water and use toothpastes with neem, coconut or oregano oil instead of fluoride.
3. Perfluorinated Chemicals (PFC). These chemicals are everywhere in the environment but are common in non-

stick cookware and stain-resistant fabrics. Consider enamel-coated cookware and natural fabrics.

4. Bisphenol A (BPA). Plastics are the main source of this chemical. Avoid cooking or storing food and water in plastics that contain BPA.

5. Perchlorate. This substance, the main component of rocket fuel, has been found in drinking water. Be sure to use filtered water whenever possible.

6. Pesticides, fungicides, and organochlorine pesticides. These are used in vegetables and fruits that are not labeled organic. They are known to cause hypothyroidism (low thyroid). Focus on buying organically raised produce and food products.

7. Make up and personal care products. These products are loaded with chemicals that are known to disrupt the function of the endocrine system. Seek out cleaner products that are organic and devoid of known endocrine disrupting chemicals.

Stress and Thyroid Function

Mental and emotional stress affects your entire body including your thyroid gland. Specifically, when you are under stress, the adrenal glands secrete the hormones cortisol and adrenaline, and when in excess both negatively affect your thyroid gland and thyroid hormone levels. Here are two main examples, and each are described below.

1. Cortisol and epinephrine/norepinephrine (adrenaline) increases reverse T3 (rT3). Cortisol and adrenaline are the main stress hormones. When under stress, these adrenal hormones increase and begin to convert T4 to inactive Reverse T3 (rT3). If inactive rT3 levels are high, then the

metabolism lowers and symptoms of hypothyroidism (low thyroid) occur.

For those who are on thyroid hormone treatment, an increase in medication dose can often push past the elevated rT3 and help relieve symptoms. But this strategy does not help everyone, or only helps to an extent. The key to better health for many patients with elevated rT3 is to lower stress. This is best accomplished by learning to identify what causes stress for you, how to lower it, and how to control your stress response. And a comprehensive medical approach to thyroid treatment must also focus on the health of the adrenal gland.

2. Cortisol decreases TSH. Stress lowers TSH. On the surface, this may sound good. Remember that an elevated TSH is often indicative of hypothyroidism (low thyroid). So if cortisol is lowering TSH, we may assume that the hypothyroid condition is being corrected. But for many people, this is not the case. In fact, long-term stress, with long-term high levels of cortisol, will continually lower TSH and not allow the thyroid to adequately make thyroid hormones, such as T4 and T3. This hinders the ability of many low thyroid patients to get the proper diagnosis. Most doctors only look at the TSH value to make their decisions to prescribe thyroid hormone medication.

Cortisol may also be hindering the ability for TSH to be produced by the pituitary gland therefore, the levels are lowered, making it look like the thyroid is fine. If the stress can be removed, the thyroid may or may not be able to adequately make thyroid hormone in the future.

Manage Your Stress, Manage Your Thyroid

The thyroid gland also represents self-expression, speaking your truth. One of the sources of pain for all humans in this world is avoiding what we really want to say and how we truly want to express ourselves. A poor interpretation, and lack of management of stress, often lead to irrational beliefs and stifles our ability to express the self in a complete way. Your entire body, including your thyroid gland, will not function at its optimum under these circumstances.

We believe that managing stress, rather than simply seeking to avoid it, is one key answer to the busy world we all find ourselves in. Everyone has his or her own ideas about stress. Your interpretation of the stress in your life is yours and yours alone. This you do have control over. The interpretation of stress involves choice. The regular practice of meditation and honest internal reflection, exercise or deep breathing may be the ways in which you've learned to thrive within your stress—rather than simply survive. Living well with stress is the key to growth. It is also one of the key reasons someone practices meditation. Meditation should teach you how to move and function within the world with the qualities of ease and grace, no matter the circumstances. How a person responds to stress is what defines character. Avoiding or being successful at living with stress has nothing to do with a person's true character and everything to do with just a basic need to survive. Do not seek to be a martyr. If you can remove yourself from situations that are unhealthy, that do not serve you, then you should—but then go even further and take steps to see the big picture and then let go.

Meditation has been subjected to the rigors of science in many ways, revealing multiple positive affects on the body. As we have already seen, the stress hormone cortisol, when in excess, negatively affects the thyroid gland and thyroid hormones. Regular meditation has the direct ability to lower and balance cortisol levels, benefitting your thyroid gland. Studies have also shown meditation easing depression, anxiety, and mood disorders. Meditation enhances mental performance and improves the ability to cope with stressful situations. People who meditate have been found to perform better on tasks that induce "deadline" stress.

We encourage the regular practice of meditation for you. Getting started is easy. Five minutes a day can do wonders. There are many resources available to you, so plan to make it a part of your regular routine. Meditation is one of the best ways to help your thyroid gland.

Exercise and Your Thyroid

Your body is designed to move! It is an inevitable fact of life... physical movement! When you are in control of your physiology, body movements dictate how your internal nature expresses itself. Physical activity stimulates hormones, the body's actual chemical messengers, to do exactly what it needs to do. One of the best forms of exercise we have found for our patients is high intensity, short duration exercise. There are three main types of exercise: light intensity, moderate intensity, and high intensity. The easiest way to distinguish them is based on your ability to speak during the exercise. During light intensity exercise or activities, you can easily hold a conversation with little to no straining. While engaging in moderate intensity exercise, you can still hold a conversation, but with some level of difficulty. High intensity exercise makes it almost impossible to talk, especially when performing at an all out maximum.

Patients often report that no matter how much exercise they do on a regular basis, it is hard to lose as much weight as when they first started the exercise program. This certainly can be from an underactive thyroid and other hormone imbalances, but often, it is the excessive amounts of cardio exercise that prevents losing more body fat. When you continue doing cardiovascular exercise to excess for weight loss, your body becomes more efficient at burning fat. Maybe this sounds exactly like what you want. But "efficiency" in this case refers to the body's way of actually preserving fat.

High intensity, short duration exercise actually stimulates the thyroid gland to produce more thyroid hormone, increasing overall metabolic rate. It also trains the body to become a fat-burning machine. This type of exercise is more efficient and it saves time. With an exercise routine that is less time consuming, you can get a more balanced, muscular, strong, and lean body that is more efficient at burning fat. This type of exercise boosts thyroid health, improves metabolism, lowers inflammation throughout the body which protects joints, muscles, and internal organs. It also lowers insulin resistance, which protects against diabetes, improves cardiovascular health, and gives the individual an improved sense of mental and emotional well-being.

Here are four ways to get you started in the right direction with an exercise plan.

1. You can do different movements that you find interesting and fun. Almost any movement can be done with high intensity and for a short duration. Remember that *intensity* of the movement is the key. For example:
   a. Sprinting/walking
   b. Stationary bike
   c. Jumping Jacks

     d. Jumping rope

     e. Weight training

2. With weight training, use compound movements that utilize as many joints in the exercise as possible, such as squats or overhead presses. Then, you can also incorporate hybrid movements by combining traditional exercise movements into one exercise, such as a squat combined with arm curls. This also has the added benefit of taking familiar, routine movements and making them fresh and fun.

3. To keep the intensity up, alternate between all out exertion of your chosen exercise and then recovery. Here's how:

     a. Beginners: (new to this type of exercise) Exert yourself for 30 seconds in your exercise of choice, then recover for 120 seconds. Repeat this six to eight times.

     b. Intermediate: (after training for about one month) Exert for 30 seconds, then recover for 90 seconds. Repeat this eight to 10 times.

     c. Advanced: (three months or more of regular training) Exert for 30 seconds, then recover for 60-90 seconds. Repeat eight to 10 times.

4. Keep your exercise time to 40 minutes or less. In fact, when you first start utilizing high intensity exercise, 10 to 20 minutes can be extremely beneficial. Remember to warm up and cool down before and after your exercise, and include light stretching once you are warmed up and at the end of the routine. You only need to exercise two to four times per week.

There are multiple factors that go into any good exercise program. Joint stability, general flexibility, overall stamina and cardiac fitness all need to be considered. The first step for most patients is to consider a competent personal trainer to guide you towards safely achieving your fitness goals. The ThyroZone system will provide you with an appropriate referral to a fitness professional.

Optimal Thyroid Hormone Medication

The ThyroZone system focuses on your unique needs, not just for your thyroid, but for your entire body and mind through proper hormonal management and a focus on your metabolic rate. When it comes to your thyroid, you need the best type of thyroid medications and medical tools to super charge both your thyroid and your body.

NDT (Natural Desiccated Thyroid) (Nature Throid®)

It is important to understand that your thyroid medication is a *hormone* medication. Thyroid medication is Hormone Replacement Therapy (HRT)–specific to thyroid hormone. You'll want to make sure you have the best form of thyroid hormone replacement medication available. This is typically Natural Desiccated Thyroid (NTD) medication such as Nature Throid® or Armour®, or at least a product that contains the active thyroid hormone called T3.

NDT comes from pig thyroid glands that under specific conditions have been desiccated or dried and standardized to contain specific amounts of thyroid hormone. This type of thyroid hormone treatment is the preferred approach in the ThyroZone system because it helps almost everyone, particularly once the optimal dose is found. Some patients have been prescribed NDT such as Armour® in the past, and it did not work. This was not necessarily because of the product itself, but most likely due to a dose that was insufficient to help with the symptoms. Once patients receive appropriate doses of the same product they had before, they experience relief.

Not many medications have such a long track record as NDT. It has been around for so long because it has helped and continues to help countless patients. In fact, NDT is one of the first true hormone replacement medications; it was used at the birth of the endocrinology field in the late 19th century and was used in one form or another historically for thousands of years.

NDT is highly effective in helping you to feel your best because it has all the hormones produced by the thyroid gland, and not just isolated singular hormones such as the medication Synthroid®. NDT contains T4 and the active thyroid hormone T3. The T3 content is one of the principle reasons patients will experience relief from their signs and symptoms. T3 packs a punch to the body's metabolism.

And, NDT has even more secrets. NDT is unique because it contains small amounts of the remaining thyroid hormones, T2, T1, thyroglobulin, and calcitonin. T2 has some limited metabolic activity and T1 acts as a building block to create active thyroid hormones such as T3. Calcitonin is also found in NDT in small amounts and is a hormone important to shuttle calcium from the blood into the bones, which in turn increases bone density. Another component of NDT is thyroglobulin, the main protein within the thyroid gland that helps to produce thyroid hormone.

This full array of hormones found in NDT makes it a more synergistic product. As you can see, NDT is a more successful treatment because this combination and the interaction of all its hormones improves its effectiveness.

In the book, *The Hormone Zone*, there is considerable detail explaining why so many doctors do not use NDT and instead almost exclusively use Synthroid®, Levoxyl®, or their generic forms (levothyroxine). You would think that the answer would be because the doctors believe those medications work better for the patient, and they likely believe this on the surface, but there are deeper reasons for their beliefs.

The simple reasons are money and politics. Synthroid® is a multi-billion dollar medication and the manufacturers of this medication fund the endocrinology medical specialty. This perspective funnels down to the general practitioner who is then persuaded and made to believe that synthetic thyroid medication is the best to use.

Another reason that NDT is not chosen by the average doctor is born from a massive misconception that forms of NDT such as Armour® or Nature Throid® are inconsistent in potency, while synthetic thyroid medications such as Synthroid® are consistent. This is not completely true.

First, it is important to note that the active thyroid hormones in *any* preparation are unstable in light, temperature, air, or humidity. These conditions can lead to issues with any batch of thyroid medication. The truth is that the synthetic thyroid medication called levothyroxine (Synthroid®) has been recalled 10 times from 1990 to 1997 and as recently in 2012 Synthroid® was recalled for batch inconsistencies. Armour® had a very small recall in 2005, but has had no issues since. Armour® reformulated in 2009 and there was a brief time where you could not get Armour®. Nature Throid®, made by RLC Labs, the product that we generally use for our patients, has *never* been recalled for hormone inconsistencies of any of its batches. They have been involved in the manufacturing of NDT since the 1930s.

One final reason doctors will not use NDT is from their parroted misconception that NDT has a ratio of T4 and T3 thyroid hormones that is inconsistent with the natural amounts of T4 and T3 found in the body. Here is an excerpt from the book *The Hormone Zone* explaining the details behind why this misconception is false. It is a little technical but we believe it is worth putting it here for you to read, question and discuss with us, or your health care professional:

> "The common argument against the use of desiccated thyroid hormone such as Nature Throid® is that the ratio of T4 to T3 of 4:1 within the medication is not physiologic for a human being. The opposition explains that humans have serum blood concentration ratios of T4 to T3 of 85.8 mcg and T4 to about 1.3 mcg of T3 or 65:1 which illustrates in their minds why T3 and desiccated thyroid hormone should not be used for hypothyroidism. But here are two facts regarding thyroid hormone physiology that they continue to ignore, even in the journals. One, production rates of T4 from the thyroid gland are 130 nmol/day/70kg body weight which equates exactly to 101.4 mcg (conversion rate for T4 is 1 nmol = 0.78 mcg) and T3 is 48 nmol/day/70kg which equates to 31.2 mcg (conversion rate for T3 is 1 nmol = 0.65 mcg), which is a ratio of T4:T3 of 3.25 to 1, far closer to the 4:1 ratio found in desiccated thyroid hormone. Two, the clearance rate of T3 from the blood is approximately twenty times more rapid than T4, which means that T3, the active form of thyroid hormone, will often be lower in the blood than T4 because it is busy doing its job at the cellular level."

After treating thousands of patients with NDT and specifically Nature Throid®, we are convinced that it is one of the best ways to help you get the relief you have always wanted. However, there are options to NDT, and the ThyroZone system will help guide you towards the best form of thyroid hormone with an optimum dose for your situation.

Dosing for NDT is in a range as broad as one-half grain to as much as six grains. *The average effective dose is from two to four grains daily.* The best dose is based on a multitude of factors, all described in this book. The most effective dose for you is one that is most effective at relieving your signs and symptoms. The best dose is not determined for you simply by blood work lab results.

Plain T3 Therapy

T3 or liothyronine is the active form of thyroid hormone. This is found in products containing NDT (Nature Throid® or Armour Thyroid®). Medications such as Cytomel, or its generic form, liothyronine, are technically synthetic because they're isolated and produced in a lab. However, liothyronine is still considered bioidentical so do not worry about the synthetic nature of it.

Natural is best, but only if it is also bioidentical in molecular shape. Synthetic hormones are not necessarily the wrong type, as long as they are bioidentical in molecular shape.

In certain cases of low metabolism, utilizing synthetic T3 medications are very helpful and effective. Some patients will not respond to NDT and will need plain T3. One specific condition that may require treatment with T3 instead of NDT is fibromyalgia. However, fibromyalgia patients do very well on NDT products such as Nature Throid®.

Dosing for T3 is as low as perhaps five to 10 mcg up to as high as 150 mcg daily. Average effective doses are approximately 50 to 100 mcg daily.

A Final Note on Thyroid Hormone Medication Choice

The best thyroid medication for you is the one that works. We tend to see clinically that this is NDT or at least a compounded product that contains T3. In some rare cases, patients simply can not tolerate T3 in any form, whether from NDT or the plain synthetic compounded medication. It is simply too stimulating to the body. In these cases, using plain T4 or levothyroxine, such as Synthroid®, is the best choice. The ThyroZone system honors the uniqueness of the individual patient and will help to determine exactly what is best for you.

Use of LDN in Hashimoto's and Grave's Diseases

Naltrexone is an FDA-approved medication at 50 mg that functions as an opiate antagonist. That is, it's normally used in treating addiction to opiate drugs such as heroin or morphine. A New York neurophysician and internist named Bernard Bihari, M.D., worked with naltrexone extensively in the 1980s and discovered that low doses of the medication were beneficial for autoimmune conditions such as Multiple Sclerosis and Crohn's Disease. During that time, others studied the medication and indeed found benefit for many autoimmune conditions. Recently, in the past decade, there has been a global rebirth of its use. Physicians and scientists from around the world are seeing the benefits of this simple medication for autoimmune disease, psychiatric conditions such as autism, bariatric (weight loss) settings, and inflammatory autoimmune conditions such as Rheumatoid Arthritis, and much more.

Naltrexone has two different isomers, or chemical shapes, in the mixture of the medication. One shape stimulates the opioid cell receptors for addiction treatment; the other shape stimulates and binds to the cell receptors on immune cells. Naltrexone has the ability to stimulate immune cells and reduce inflammatory elements known as cytokines, that are involved in many diseases, including Hashimoto's thyroiditis and Grave's disease. We have found this simple medication can be very helpful at reducing the inflammatory response and the autoimmune response. It is another tool in helping to regulate the immune system and lessen the attack that is occurring in the thyroid gland, thereby reducing autoantibodies such as Anti-TPO and Anti-TG.

LDN Dosing

The dosing for LDN is approximately 1.5 to 4.5 mg daily, with the 4.5 mg dose being the most widely accepted and currently the one that we use most often in the ThyroZone system . The dose is kept low initially and gradually increased to 4.5 mg over a few weeks.

LDN Side Effects

This medication is extremely safe with minimal problems. There are some potential gastrointestinal disturbances but starting with a low dose helps to avoid this. Nighttime doses can induce vivid dreams or even insomnia. We have not seen many gastrointestinal disturbances with our patients, but occasionally we have reports of vivid dreams that are troublesome. In this case, we simply switch the dosing to daytime to avoid this problem.

A positive "side effect" of LDN that many patients report is an improved sense of well being. This is due in part to the improvement in endorphins, chemicals that induce this sense of well being. This is one of the reasons many psychiatrists have found profound benefit with its use.

ThyroZone Research on LDN

We are currently conducting observational research on the use of LDN with Hashimoto's thyroiditis and its ability to lower autoantibodies such as anti-TPO and anti-TG. Data is being tracked including blood work analysis and patient outcomes. We are reporting our findings to the LDN Research Trust in an ongoing effort to spread awareness of this effective medication.

How to Monitor Your Progress

Once your diagnosis and treatment are established, you will be on the road to recovery, and, optimization. At first, the focus will be on digging you out of the hole, and that could take a little bit of time...normally a few months. But once you are above ground and running, you will need to have ongoing intricate monitoring, dose adjustment, and maintenance of your metabolism.

Over time, your personal therapy may need to be modified in order to maintain your results. Humans are not static beings, so things change from time to time, and the ThyroZone system will be there to observe those changes and make quick refinements to keep you on track.

Symptom Questionnaires

You've seen the questionnaires. Now you're ready to use these questionnaires in an ongoing way by answering the questions over the course of time. Be sure to compare each questionnaire you complete with previous questionnaires. Did symptoms improve? If not, then it is important to consider adjusting your treatment plan, whether by an increased thyroid hormone dose, or addressing something else that still remains. The Zulewski's Clinical Score for hypothyroidism (low thyroid) should be less than five. The Wayne's Hyperthyroid Score for hyperthyroidism (high thyroid) should be less than 11.

Some of the additional questions to ask yourself and your doctor along the course of managing your treatment are:

1. Have my thyroid symptoms improved from month to month?
2. Based on the results of my ThyroFlex and/or my ReeVue®, is my metabolic rate optimized? Is it slow or fast?
3. Have I been taking my thyroid hormone medication on a consistent basis?
4. How are my stress levels?
5. How am I handling the stress that I have in my life? Has my adrenal health been tested and treated yet?
6. Am I improving my diet for optimized thyroid and metabolic recovery?
7. Do I have food allergies such as gluten intolerance?
8. Am I skipping meals?
9. Do I have symptoms of hypoglycemia (low blood sugar)?
10. Have I been taking all of the appropriate supplements related to my thyroid condition and metabolism?

11. Are there additional supportive supplements that can help with the symptoms that have not improved yet?
12. Am I exercising appropriately?
13. Is my exercise too little or too much?
14. Am I exercising in a specific way that actually positively affects my metabolic rate?
15. Are all of my other hormones balanced yet?

Depending on the answers to these additional questions, you can assess if you have arrived or not yet reached your health goals. Be sure to continue asking any and all other questions you may have while on your road to recovery and optimization.

Blood Work

Now that we understand which labs are important, let's explore each thyroid lab parameter and discuss the *optimal* ranges for each one. Each value listed should be the minimal goal for each patient. Remember that these optimal values reflect someone undergoing treatment.

Thyroid Hormones

TSH. For the patient with hypothyroidism (low thyroid) and is taking thyroid hormone medication with the ThyroZone system, usually the TSH is "suppressed," showing a number that is well below the range and near zero, such as 0.01 U/mL, or even lower. This is usually, but not always, the best value for most patients to get good results when on thyroid hormone medication. Remember that the TSH does *not* tell us if you are over-stimulated or not. Your body's response tells us this. For the patient being monitored for hyperthyroidism (high thyroid), the goal of therapy is to keep the TSH above 0.30 U/mL.

Total T4. greater than 8 ug/dL but less than 12.5 ug/dL.

Free T4. greater than 1.2 ug/dL but less than 2.0 ug/dL.

Total T3. greater than 100 ug/dL but less than 200 ug/dL.

Free T3. greater than 3.0 pg/mL but less than 4.8 pg/mL.

Reverse T3.: less than 13 ng/dL.

Note: If Reverse T3 (RT3) is very elevated, particularly greater than 20 ng/dL, then some form of stress is often the culprit. It could be situational stress as well as dieting, both of which increase stress and the hormone cortisol, which in turn will increase RT3. We have also seen the RT3 go up as the dose of thyroid hormone increases for a patient, so it's not necessarily always an issue of stress. This speaks to the fact that as thyroid hormone elevates in the body, a natural response to prevent over-stimulation to thyroid hormone would be to produce more RT3, the inactive form of thyroid hormone.

Antibodies

Anti-TPO. < 34 IU/mL. Essentially, this value should be as low as possible.

Anti-TG. < 40 IU/mL. Essentially, this value should be as low as possible.

TSI. the TSI Index should be less than 1.3. Again, this value should be as low as possible.

A note for blood testing: Be sure to avoid taking your thyroid hormone medication for at least 24 hours before your serum blood tests. Taking the thyroid hormone too soon around the time of the lab will show a transient rise in thyroid hormone levels.

Resting Metabolic Rate (RMR) Testing

Remember, your RMR is the calories your body burns when at rest.

ThyroFlex®

You will have routine monitoring with the ThyroFlex as you move forward with the treatment. It is important to make sure your thyroid hormone medication and your medical thyroid supplements are optimizing your metabolism.

The ThyroFlex measures reflex speed in milliseconds. The higher the value, the slower your reflex is moving, and the slower your metabolism is moving. Here are the values:

Optimal: Your reflex speed should be between 50 and 100 ms. Satisfactory: 100 to 120 ms.

Borderline: 120 to 136 ms.

Hypothyroid (Low Thyroid): Greater than 136 ms.

Hyperthyroid (High Thyroid or a fast metabolism): Less than 50 ms.

Depending on the results of the ThyroFlex, your treatment may be adjusted. For those patients with hypothyroidism (low thyroid), the thyroid hormone dose will be gradually and carefully increased until the value improves and symptoms abate. Once you are stabilized you will have routine ThyroFlex tests throughout the year.

ReeVue® Indirect Calorimetry Testing

This test is often used in conjunction with the ThyroFlex test while you are being monitored on your thyroid hormone treatment. The optimal range for this test is +/- 5 percent. The lower the number, the slower the metabolism; the higher the number, the higher the metabolism. For those patients with hypothyroidism (low thyroid), the thyroid hormone dose will be gradually and carefully *increased* until the value improves and symptoms abate. Once you are optimized, you will have routine ReeVue® tests throughout the year.

Electrocardiogram (ECG)

Here is some specific information on what your ECG may look like if you had either low thyroid or high thyroid. It gets a little technical here, but it's a great reference. You can show the results of your ECG to your doctor to see if there are any of these abnormalities. Most ECG results will automatically report abnormal findings on the ECG readout, allowing you to reference the following potential abnormalities.

In hypothyroidism (low thyroid and low metabolism):

- Low voltage (voltage of an entire QRS complex in all limb leads ≤5 mm (millimeters) or ≤10 mm in the precordial lead)
- Prolonged QT interval >460 ms
- Bradycardia (slow heart rate < 50 beats per minute)

In hyperthyroidism (high thyroid and elevated metabolism):

- Continuous atrial fibrillation (rapid contraction of the atria only)
- Sinus tachycardia (fast heart beat > 100)
- Shortened QT interval of < 300 ms (milliseconds)
- PR interval prolongation > 200 ms

The results of an ECG can be from many conditions that are genetic and do not necessarily reflect an influence with thyroid hormone. The use of the ECG is considered in the entire clinical presentation. If one of these ECG parameters are abnormal but no other signs or symptoms of overstimulation to thyroid hormone exist, then it is not necessarily the thyroid hormone causing the issue.

After treating thousands of patients with adequate doses of thyroid hormone that often suppress the TSH, we have never had any issues with the thyroid hormone dosing being related to an abnormal ECG or even comprehensive cardiac workups that include stress tests and other advanced cardiac tests. However, an ECG can show when someone has an unrelated cardiac abnormality that warrants a referral to a cardiologist. This is always important and the ThyroZone system is designed to ensure safe medical care by making referrals to other specialists when needed. Finally, the ECG is used on a routine basis to verify that your cardiac function is adequate enough to handle the stimulation provided by the thyroid hormone.

Other Monitoring Parameters Used in ThyroZone

Blood Pressure. This simple test can produce accurate monitoring of body changes. The blood pressure monitor will also be able to provide an accurate digital readout of your heart rate. Blood pressure should be no higher than 120/80 mm mercury. Often, hypothyroid and patients with low metabolisms will have very low blood pressure readings, such as a typical 90/60, without the physical fitness to justify it.

Heart Rate. An average heart rate is about seventy-two beats per minute. Many patients with low metabolisms will have a heart rate in the low sixties or even lower, without the fitness to warrant it. If your heart rate starts to elevate into the nineties, and you are taking thyroid medication, your dose could be too high. When being monitored on thyroid hormone medication, it is important to distinguish between the effects of stress and hypoglycemia (low blood sugar) when considering elevated heart rate.

Body weight. Changes in overall body weight can be used to determine improvement, particularly if you are overweight. Rapid reductions in weight can be suggestive of excessive thyroid hormone medication or a hypermetabolic state. Your weight will be closely monitored while on the ThyroZone system.

Body fat percentage. Body fat percentage is a far more accurate measurement of weight loss goals. Utilizing a Bioelectrical Impedance Analysis (BIA) body fat analysis machine can help to monitor how you are improving. It is better to look at your body fat percentage and relative muscle mass versus your body weight alone. Optimal body fat percentages vary based on age and gender. In general, women should seek to keep their body fat percentage from 25-30 percent or lower. Men should range from 20-25 percent body fat or less.

Waist-to-Hip ratio. This ratio helps determine your level of health and fitness and progress while on the ThyroZone system. It is also a predictor of disease, particularly diabetes. The waist is measured with a tape measure at the smallest circumference of the natural waist, usually just above the navel. The hip circumference may likewise be measured at its widest part of the buttocks or hip. To calculate your ratio, divide waist inch count by your hip inch size. A waist-to-hip ratio of 0.7 for women and 0.9 for men have been shown to correlate strongly with general health and decreased tendency towards metabolic syndrome and diabetes. The normal waist-to-hip ratio for women is 0.7 to 0.8 and 0.9 to 0.99 for men.

Thyroid Dose Adjustments for Hypothyroid Patients

When you are first put on thyroid hormone medication, the dose will be slowly increased over time to the most effective dose that relieves your symptoms and enhances your metabolic rate. You will normally start on about one half to one grain of NDT hormone medication and increase by half-grain increments every week until you reach about two to three grains daily.

During the course of treatment on thyroid hormone medication and the entire ThyroZone system, it will be necessary to adjust the dose of your thyroid hormone medication to improve the clinical response. Sometimes up or down. Keep in mind that the *average* dose for NDT is between two and four grains (approximately 120 to 240 mg) daily. Some patients need less, some more. The goal is to closely monitor progress and adjust as needed.

Signs and Symptoms of Overstimulation

Wayne's Hyperthyroid Index (WHI) provides a comprehensive analysis of the traditional signs and symptoms of being in a "thyrotoxic" state. That means the body tissues are over-stimulated by thyroid hormone. It is always worth repeating, for the sake of continued clarification, that your thyroid labs do *not* necessarily indicate that you are either hyperthyroid or thyrotoxic. Your body tissues and metabolic rate provide the best measurement of this potential issue.

When you are over-stimulated from thyroid hormone, it feels as if you have had too much coffee or caffeine. In general, you are anxious, jittery, shaky, sweating, with heart palpitations and an increased heart rate.

Troubleshooting Overstimulation to Thyroid Hormone Medication

As your thyroid hormone medication dose gradually increases, you may have any of the symptoms described above. If you do experience these at any time and are uncertain as to why they are there, simply *stop* your thyroid hormone medication completely for three days and lower the dose of thyroid medication back down to the dose that did not cause any problems. Also, call your prescribing doctor immediately and report your situation. Generally, there is nothing to be overly concerned about. The half life of the T3 portion of your medication is three days, and after stopping the medication, your metabolism rate will quickly lower.

Please be very diligent with communicating to your doctor about what you are experiencing.

The Top Seven Reasons for Over-stimulation by Thyroid Hormone Medication

1. Hypoglycemia (low blood sugar) and skipping meals. The symptoms of hypoglycemia are virtually identical to the symptoms of overstimulation to thyroid hormone. Thyroid hormone has the ability to lower blood sugar due to increased metabolism. For patients who routinely skip meals, and for those who eat mostly carbohydrate, this could be a problem. Be sure to keep your blood sugar balanced.

2. Poor cardiovascular fitness. If you are out of shape, then the chances are greater that you will have a problem with overstimulation to thyroid medication.

3. Lack of nutritional status. If you are deficient in most nutrients, particularly B vitamins and minerals, the

odds of having an issue with overstimulation are greater. This is one of the main reasons supportive nutritional supplementation is so important.

4. You are in the middle of a "Hashimoto's Flare." This is a sudden excessive production of thyroid antibodies from an immune reaction. This is most often caused by stress, sudden illness such as bacterial or viral infections, and diet factors such as gluten and lectins.

5. Weak adrenal function and poor stress adaptability. Your adrenal glands respond to stress. If you have either elevated or low adrenal hormones, you may experience more symptoms of overstimulation to thyroid hormone. First, addressing the adrenal issues may be required before the thyroid hormone dose can be increased.

6. Sex hormone deficiency. If your sex hormones, such as estrogen and testosterone, are low and imbalanced, then there is a greater chance of having overstimulation.

7. The thyroid hormone dose needs to be lowered.

Note about over-stimulation and thyrotoxicosis in the true hyperthyroid patient: If you are experiencing any of the symptoms of overstimulation described here and in the Wayne's Hyperthyroid Index (WHI), follow the acute plan that was previously created by your doctor and call immediately.

Troubleshooting Overstimulation and Thyrotoxicosis in the True Hyperthyroid Patient

If you are diagnosed with true hyperthyroidism (high thyroid) and are not on thyroid hormone medication, then the dosing of other medications such as iodine therapy and use of Melissa officinalis will often need to be adjusted. In hyperthyroidism (high thyroid), monitoring TSH and Free T3 levels can be helpful in determining the benefits of treatment. Of course, following the symptoms laid out in the Wayne's Hyperthyroid Index (WHI) and the RMR analysis is extremely important. For example, if your TSH is still below the range, then your iodine dose and other potential medications would need to be increased until your TSH is normalized.

The main reasons why someone would not be progressing in their hyperthyroid (high thyroid) treatment would be elevated emotional and physical stress, poor diet (particularly if there are gluten and other food allergies), other hormonal imbalances such as in the adrenal and sex hormones, and poor compliance with the supportive nutritional and botanical tools prescribed.

Optimal Diet and Lifestyle

We explored a beneficial thyroid diet in Chapter 6. The details and reasoning supporting this plan are there for you. We want to inspire you to change your eating habits, and to monitor and assess your progress as you improve your diet.

As previously discussed, another important deterrent to progress is a poor stress response and making decisions that are simply not healthy. Be sure to continually ask yourself the tough questions about how you can address these factors in order to get the most out of your treatment.

Ask yourself these questions:
1. Is my diet the best it can be?
2. Am I following the recommendations set out in this book?
3. Do I really understand the medical reasoning behind the diet and stress relief recommendations?
4. What small change can I make TODAY to improve my diet?
5. What commitments can I make to my family and myself for my diet over the next 30 days?

6. Am I choosing organic produce and foods whenever possible?
7. How can I make my food preparation easier?
8. Should I consider a meal preparation service?
9. Should I seek the additional help of a nutritionist?
10. Am I taking all of the nutritional and herbal supplements suggested? If not, why?
11. Have I discussed any difficulties with the supplements with my doctor?
12. Am I avoiding as many unnecessary chemicals in my household?
13. What basic hygiene products could I replace today with something that is less toxic?
14. Have I explored healthy, less toxic versions of shampoo and cosmetics?
15. Where are my stress levels?
16. Do I really know if I am stressed?
17. Do others around me think I am not handling my stress?
18. What are my typical outward responses to stress?
19. What are my coping mechanisms?
20. Have I really followed the stress advice in this book?
21. Do I have a good support group?
22. Do I surround myself with people who support me and help to lower my stress?
23. Should I consider the help of a professional counselor?

Be sure to ask your doctor is you have need of guidance on any of these questions. Seek out those who can guide you and serve you. There are always answers and there are always options. Both Dr. Bosch and Dr. Robinson are here to help you.

8

A Brief Introduction to The Hormone Zone© and Putting It All Together

The Hormone Zone® is a book title, a cutting-edge Medical Practice *and* the balanced intersection of all your hormonal systems. This hormonal intersection is from the place that all health pivots. The endocrine system, with all of its hormonal messages and communications, is where true health begins.

To achieve comprehensive hormonal care for your thyroid health, we must consider a broad comprehensive view that covers a multitude of hormones. There are over 80 hormones in your body, performing multiple functions all the time, literally keeping you alive and well. It is an ongoing dance. And you must be willing to dance with them, help and guide them when necessary.

Part of the ThyroZone® System is the intimate relationship

with The Hormone Zone® System. The Hormone Zone® is the quintessential and premiere medical practice that focuses on complete hormonal balance.

The two of us, John A. Robinson and Cristina Romero-Bosch, are naturopathic medical doctors who bring over two decades of combined experience with hormone replacement therapy and health optimization. At The Hormone Zone®, we strive towards four key ideals:

Comprehensive Hormonal Care

Optimization of Health

Peak Performance in Life

Taking Health to The Next Level

We endeavor to bring you to your best self. We never settle, so neither should you.

Sex Hormones and Your Thyroid

The first things we will assess in our comprehensive approach to your hormone balance are your sex hormones. The main sex hormones produced by the ovaries are estrogen, testosterone, and progesterone. The testicles produce principally testosterone. In both men and women, these vital hormones influence sexual development and growth, brain power and mood balance, memory and mental drive, muscle and bone growth and maintenance, immune balance, plus a feeling of being alive and at your best.

The thyroid influences estrogen, testosterone, and progesterone levels; they influence the thyroid as well. One system is strengthening the other. As men and women age, and sex hormones start to decline and the thyroid attempts to pick up the slack. Depending on the nutritional state of the thyroid and other environmental factors, the thyroid may not be able to keep up. In fact, this is a typical outcome for women when they first enter menopause; thyroid dysfunction often coincides with the transition to menopause.

Many of the relationships with thyroid function and sex hormones are extremely important. Here is a summary of some of the various effects of sex hormones on thyroid function and how it potentially minimizes or increases the activity of thyroid hormone.

Estradiol increases Thyroid Binding Globulin (TBG). Thyroid Binding Globulin is a protein that binds up thyroid hormone in the body. The higher TBG is in your body, the lower the benefits of thyroid hormone. One of the concerns about estrogen replacement therapy for women is that it lowers the effectiveness of thyroid hormone in the body by increasing TBG. But with the proper balance of testosterone, it should not be an issue because testosterone *lowers* TBG.

Testosterone decreases TBG. A balance of both estrogen and testosterone for women will help keep TBG lowered and keep thyroid hormone readily available. This action of *lowering* TBG is another reason why testosterone tends to help with increasing metabolic rate by indirectly enhancing thyroid hormone availability.

Progesterone likely decreases TBG. Less is known about progesterone's effects on thyroid hormone. Progesterone is important particularly for women in helping to balance the physiological effects of estrogen.

Estradiol lowers TSH. When women first enter perimenopause and eventually menopause, which is accompanied by lowered estrogen, it is very common to develop hypothyroidism (low thyroid), and an elevation in TSH. Restoring the estrogen levels will help to lower TSH, partially relieving the low thyroid state.

Estradiol increases T4 and T3. Estrogen also directly stimu-lates the thyroid gland to produce more thyroid hormone, which contributes to lowering TSH.

Here are examples of how the thyroid benefits sex hormone production by stimulating the testicles or the ovaries.

T3 increases the sensitivity of Luteinizing Hormone (LH). LH is a pituitary hormone, just like TSH, but stimulates the testicles or ovaries to make sex hormones. The active thyroid hormone T3 has the benefit of making LH more sensitive on the testicles and ovaries, therefore increasing testosterone and estrogen produc-tion.

Low thyroid leads to enlarged and cystic ovaries. Thyroid hormone positively influences a woman's ovaries, keeping them functioning optimally and clear of waste products that can lead to cysts. Many female gynecological conditions that seem to be all about ovarian function really stem from a thyroid condition.

Sometimes sex hormones are deficient or respond in weak ways because of a hypothyroid (low thyroid) condition. We have had a number of patients, particularly younger, pre- and peri-menopausal women, who have gynecological issues such as men-strual irregularities that were not simply an "ovarian" issue, but a thyroid hormone issue. Correcting the thyroid condition helps with the sex hormone condition, without having to replace the sex hormones or consider taking the synthetic birth control pills, which is a typical gynecological approach for menstrual irregu-larities.

If your sex hormones are deficient, such as estrogen, proges-terone, and testosterone, your thyroid will suffer. Part of your comprehensive Hormone Zone® assessment will include blood tests, a physical exam, and questionnaires to determine sex hormone deficiencies.

Based on the results of your assessment, there are two possible

treatment options: hormone restoring and hormone replacement. "Hormone restoring" means reestablishing the body's
natural ability to produce hormone, when it is possible. For
younger patients, mostly those under 50 years of age, hormone
levels and function can be restored by stimulating the body and
the endocrine glands to produce hormones through nutritional
and herbal methods.

Eventually, it becomes important to get a little more help.
"Hormone replacement" means introducing natural, bioidentical prescription hormones to replace what the body has difficulty
producing on its own, despite natural encouragement with nutritional, herbal, and glandular support.

At the Hormone Zone©, we consider which of the two methods
are of most benefit for you. Often both are used simultaneously
to give you the best results.

Hormone Replacement Options at The Hormone Zone©

Subcutaneous Hormone Pellets. A superior way to introduce
consistent levels of natural, bioidentical estrogen and testosterone for both men and women, keeping your hormone levels
consistent, and you feeling your best for up to six months. A time-
tested medical therapy, Hormone Pellets have been used successfully since 1937 in Europe and 1939 in the U.S. In a simple five
minute procedure, a Hormone Zone© trained physician inserts
subcutaneous hormone pellets under your skin. As short as 24
hours later, you are beginning to experience relief and benefit.
This is a profound therapy that both Dr. Robinson and Dr. Bosch
offer as industry leaders, having treated thousands of patients in
this therapy.

Testosterone Injections. At The Hormone Zone©, we have

developed a system of keeping the levels of testosterone consistent with using a subcutaneous injection in the abdomen twice
weekly. This can be done for both men and women, although a
majority of men come to us for this treatment. Along with proper
ongoing assessment of hormone levels and additional hormone
support with Human Chorionic Gonadotropin (HCG) to support
testicular health and function, men can expect superior hormone
replacement results.

Be sure to explore our website at www.hormone-zone.com
to determine if you have a sex hormone imbalance and how our
unique therapies can help you.

Adrenals and Your Thyroid

Stress is an inevitable part of life. When managed correctly it
becomes an ally that serves you, drives you towards your highest
and best personal goals, even your goals of achieving peace and
calm. But when stress is not handled correctly, it can overwhelm
your ability to recover and lead to adrenal dysfunction, which
ultimately causes your health to suffer.

At The Hormone Zone®, we will assist you in understanding
your stress, managing the adrenal hormones released during
stress, and teach you to use them to your advantage.

Your adrenal glands are small glands that sit on top of your
kidneys, producing many hormones necessary to sustain life.
These adrenal hormones include cortisol, adrenaline (epineph-
rine/norepinephrine), DHEA, aldosterone, androstenedione,
estrogen, testosterone, and progesterone. All adrenal hormones
respond to the input of stress. If you have adrenal dysfunction
and your adrenal glands are either overproducing or underpro-
ducing hormones, then you can have a long list of problems. Your
thyroid and sex hormones will suffer also.

Here are the important ways your adrenals—and the cortisol they produce—affect your ovaries or testicles and your thyroid. Cortisol is secreted in excess during stress. When there is an excess of cortisol, it blocks the ability of your estrogen and testosterone to be produced at either the ovaries or the testicles. Cortisol also blocks the ability of sex hormones to travel from the blood into the cell, where all the action lies. This causes disruption of hormone that can lead to disturbed or painful menstrual cycles, skipping cycles, and a host of other sex hormone problems including fatigue and irritability.

Cortisol, in excess, will prevent the active form of thyroid hormone, T3, from getting absorbed by the cells by decreasing T3 receptors. Excess cortisol will also convert active T3 into the inactive thyroid hormone called rT3 or "reverse" T3. This further lowers your metabolism and harms the body.

The adrenal/thyroid axis is one of the most important hormone conversations in your body. The adrenals and the thyroid are two vital players. Adrenal hormones stimulate the thyroid gland, and thyroid hormones stimulate and regulate the adrenal glands. Working to keep both of them optimized is the key to helping each of them.

Here are some of the general effects of adrenal hormones on thyroid function:

Cortisol and epinephrine/norepinephrine (adrenaline) increases Reverse T3 (rT3). Cortisol and adrenaline are the main stress hormones. When under stress, these adrenal hormones increase and begin to influence the conversion of T4 into active T3 and instead convert T4 to inactive rT3. If inactive rT3 levels are high, then the metabolism lowers and symptoms of hypothyroidism (low thyroid) ensue, despite good levels of T4 and active T3.

Cortisol decreases TSH. Stress lowers TSH but remember

that an elevated TSH is often indicative of hypothyroidism (low thyroid). So if cortisol is lowering TSH, one may assume that the hypothyroid condition is being corrected. But for many, this is not the case. In fact, long-term stress, with long term high levels of cortisol, will continually lower TSH and not allow the thyroid to adequately make thyroid hormone, such as T4 and T3. This will hinder the ability for many low thyroid patients to get the proper diagnosis because most doctors only look at the TSH value to decide whether or not to prescribe thyroid hormone medication.

Cortisol may also be hindering the ability for TSH to be produced by the pituitary and therefore the levels are lowered, making it look like the thyroid is fine. If the stress can be removed, the thyroid may or may not be able to adequately make thyroid hormone in the future.

If your adrenal glands are in a dysfunctional state and your ongoing stress is unmanaged, preventing you from continuing to perform at your best, then your thyroid health is compromised. The goal of our comprehensive approach to hormone balance is to help you stabilize adrenal function and improve stress management.

Adrenal Repair Options at The Hormone Zone©

Adrenal Support. The first step in your journey will be to establish an exact diagnosis of what is going on. We determine your unique adrenal issue with specific salivary and urine testing, that shows how your adrenal glands function throughout the entire day and evening. With this specific information a unique nutritional and herbal approach can be provided to solve dysfunction. At times, a prescription for natural bioidentical cortisol (hydrocortisone) will be provided. When cortisol levels lower, fatigue, poor immunity, anxiety, depression, food cravings, and much more, can become prevalent. Hydrocortisone can be a life-altering solution for many people.

Mitochondrial Support. Mitochondria are the cellular powerhouses that supply the body with energy. Their impairment is often implicated in adrenal dysfunction, Chronic Fatigue Syndrome, Fibromyalgia, and thyroid disease. Cutting-edge testing can reveal if you are suffering from a mitochondrial disorder, and through proper nutritional and lifestyle support, optimal function can be restored.

Learn more at our website, www.hormone-zone.com, to determine if you have adrenal dysfunction and how our unique therapies can help you.

Insulin and Your Thyroid

The hormone most responsible for ensuring proper balance of your blood sugar (glucose) is insulin. It is also the largest culprit in weight gain. Part of your comprehensive hormonal assessment with The Hormone Zone® will include a close examination of your insulin and other parameters that are associated with an imbalance in this system.

Excessive carbohydrates lead to insulin resistance, the condition where cells no longer respond effectively to insulin and blood sugar elevates. This scenario is the hallmark of diabetes. Insulin resistance is an epidemic in this country; nearly 86 million people have the condition, to some varying degree.

Low thyroid hormone levels decrease the sensitivity of insulin on the cell, leading to fat gain (i.e. insulin resistance). One of the common symptoms of hypothyroidism (low thyroid) is weight gain. This is in part due to a lowered metabolic rate. But another factor in weight gain is due to a lack of thyroid hormone that affects insulin receptors to respond to the insulin hormone. Thyroid hormone normally helps insulin to shuttle glucose (blood sugar) into the cell. This mechanism prevents insulin resistance and diabetes.

High thyroid (hyperthyroidism) also decreases the sensitivity of insulin on the cell, paradoxically, this also leads to fat gain: Excess thyroid hormone, in a very complex process with insulin and glucose (blood sugar) both rising and falling, yields an overall result of insulin resistance. In essence, excessive thyroid hormone is over-communicating with many parts of the body, leading to high blood sugar and insulin resistance.

Too much insulin blocks the conversion of the thyroid hormone T4 to T3. Again, T3 is the active thyroid hormone, not T4. We make T4 in the thyroid gland, but it is the conversion of T4 to active T3 that helps cells to function correctly. When you ingest high amounts of carbohydrates and stimulate high levels of insulin, you prevent the conversion of T4 to T3. This can lead to a lowered metabolic rate and hypothyroidism (low thyroid).

The epidemic of insulin resistance and diabetes is on the rise in the developed world. And the intimate relationship between your diet, carbohydrate intake, and thyroid function poses a potential problem for your health. The more insulin is controlled, the easier it is to lose weight, balance mood, increase energy, prevent other problems like cardiovascular disease, and of course, thyroid disease.

Insulin Balancing Options at The Hormone Zone©

At The Hormone Zone®, we take diet and lifestyle very seriously to enhance your health and performance. We offer a medically guided diet that produces the results you expect: fat loss, muscle building, and insulin control. Upon the foundation of the proper diet, we add nutritional and botanical options with functional prescription medications that control insulin and boost your metabolism.

Diet counseling and suggestions are a cornerstone for insulin regulation and diabetes treatment. The Traditional Ancestral Diet that is described in this book is one of the general recommendations we make for patients needing to balance insulin and blood sugar. We have also had excellent benefits with our patients using a Ketogenic Diet, that focuses on a 75% fat, 20% protein, and 5% carbohydrate model. This type of diet induces profound metabolic changes that decreases body fat, lowers blood sugar and insulin, and increases energy and metabolic activity. We guide patients through this diet with routine "ketone" blood measurements. Ketones are the main element of fat burning exhaust. This process is done until they realize the metabolic benefits necessary for clinical improvement.

Be sure to explore our website at www.hormone-zone.com for the unique diet options and comprehensive approach to your insulin health.

Growth Hormone and Your Thyroid

One of the most powerful hormones in your body is human Growth Hormone (hGH). It signals growth and maturation for your entire body, and in adulthood it maintains skin integrity, and muscle and bone health. The growth hormone continues to serve a role in repairing your organs and improving brain and mood stability. And there is an intimate relationship with growth hormone and your thyroid function.

hGH controls thyroid production. In a hyperthyroid (high thyroid) state, where thyroid hormone is in excess, growth hormone has the ability to lower thyroid hormone production.

hGH increases conversion of T4 to T3. hGH increases an enzyme known as 5' deiodinase which is responsible for cleaving one iodine molecule off of the T4 hormone, converting it into the active thyroid hormone T3. This is extremely important because hGH has shown to increase metabolic rate and fat oxidation (burning), and this increase in T3 plays a role.

hGH lowers Reverse T3 (rT3). Growth hormone is also responsible for controlling the production of rT3, an inactive form of thyroid hormone that competes with active T3 and lowers metabolic rate in your cells.

Thyroid hormone enhances hGH. Here we see the complimentary effects of how thyroid hormone affects hGH, both by stimulating the production of hGH and enhancing its effects.

Just like your other hormones, growth hormone communicates with your thyroid gland and influences the function of thyroid hormone. One hormone helps the other, all moving in an intricate dance. Growth hormone is one of the most potent hormones for longevity and health, serving as the lynchpin of all other hormonal systems. When enhanced, this hormone will help your thyroid and change your life.

Growth Hormone Enhancement Options at The Hormone Zone©

Nutritional and Exercise Counseling. Amino acid therapy has been shown to enhance growth hormone production. When coupled with a diet that is focused on protein and minimized carbohydrates, growth hormone production is enhanced. Excessive fat tissue blocks the production of growth hormone, so fat loss is also key to enhancing growth hormone production.

Testosterone Replacement Therapy. Testosterone is one of the most potent stimulators of natural growth hormone production. Your comprehensive hormonal examination will include accurate assessment of testosterone levels, with the option of natural, bioidentical hormone replacement therapy.

Peptide Therapy. An advanced hormone therapy that uses special peptides that communicates with your pituitary gland to produce more Human Growth Hormone (hGH). Peptide Therapy is extremely safe and has no known side effects. This is often the starting option when a growth hormone deficiency is discovered, particularly for patients from 40 to 60 years of age. There are many different natural peptide secretagogues that we will also prescribe depending on the needs of the patient.

Human Growth Hormone Therapy. For the patient with a considerable deficiency of growth hormone and multiple signs of aging, hGH is a superior option for those patients ready to take their health to the next level, particularly those over 60 years of age.

Explore our website at www.hormone-zone.com for more information on how growth hormone enhancement can help you.

Conclusion

ThyroZone was created for you. It is a commitment to the never-ending cause for true patient-centered medicine, and the unrelenting vision for peak performance and excellent health for everyone. Dr. Robinson and Dr. Bosch share a Grand Vision for all patients suffering with thyroid disease to finally experience the natural relief and life balance they deserve. It is said that the thyroid is about speaking your truth. So let this small book be a large opportunity for you and your loved ones and the entire world to finally be heard.

The Hormone Zone© is comprehensive hormonal care, supporting your thyroid, all of your main hormone systems, and enhancing your entire life. Our unique approach to wellness and age management medicine leads the way through what is a seemingly difficult path to restored health. We welcome you and your loved ones to learn how to walk that path and experience the profound benefits of hormonal health.

Resources and References

Thyroid Resources for Patients

Thyroid Nation: http://thyroidnation.com
Stop the Thyroid Madness: http://www.stopthethyroidmadness.
    com
Hypothyroid Mom: http://hypothyroidmom.com

Thyroid Resources for Physicians

Thyroid Disease Manager: http://www.thyroidmanager.org

Chapter 1

The Hormone Zone© website, www.hormone-zone.com

Chapter 2

Thyroid Disease Manager: http://www.thyroidmanager.org
Teach Me Anatomy: http://teachmeanatomy.info/neck/viscera/
    the-thyroid-gland/

Chapter 3

"Endocrine Disrupting Chemicals: A Scientific Statement: An
    Endocrine Society Scientific Statement." Available at: https://
    www.endocrine.org/~/media/endosociety/Files/.../EDC_
    Scientific_Statement.pdf
"Worldwide Increasing Incidence of Thyroid Cancer: Update on
    Epidemiology and Risk Factors." Pellegriti, et. al. Available at:
    https://www.hindawi.com/journals/jce/2013/965212/
Statistics by Country for Thyroid disorders. Available at:
    http://www.rightdiagnosis.com/t/thyroid/stats-country.
    htm#extrapwarning
The Endocrine Society. Endocrine Facts and Figures. Hypothy-
    roidism. Available at: http://endocrinefacts.org/health-con-
    ditions/thyroid/3-hypothyroidism/
A Compilation of Iodine Research. Available at: http://iodinere-
    search.com/disease_thyroid_nodule.html

Chapter 4

"Rethinking the TSH Test: An Interview with David Derry, M.D.,
    Ph.D.: The History of Thyroid Testing, Why the TSH Test
    Needs to Be Abandoned, and the Return to Symptoms-Based
    Thyroid Diagnosis and Treatment." Available at: http://www.
    thyroid-info.com/articles/david-derry.htm

Sir Richard Bayliss, "How thyroid patients see us," British Thyroid Foundation, *BTF News*, Nos. 13-15, Summer 1995-Winter 1995.

Chapter 5

Thyroflex Testing: Explore www.thyroflex.com

Thyroid Thermography: http://www.imedpub.com/articles/ thermographic-analysis-of-thyroid-diseases-at-the-lagos- university-teachinghospital-nigeria.pdf

Kalra S, Khandelwal SK, Goyal A. Clinical scoring scales in thyroidology: A compendium. *Indian J Endocrinol Metab.* 2011 Jul; 15(Suppl 2):S89-94.

"The Differences Between the Weston A. Price Foundation Diet and The Paleo Diet." Available at: http://www.westonaprice.org/health-topics/differences- between-the-weston-a-price-foundation-diet-and-the- paleo-diet/

"The Whole Soy Story" by Dr. Kaayla Daniel. Available at: http:// www.wholesoystory.com

Sasso FC, Carbonara O, Torella R, Mezzogiorno A, Esposito V, Demagistris L, Secondulfo M, Carratu' R, Iafusco D, Cartenì M. Ultrastructural changes in enterocytes in subjects with Hashimoto's thyroiditis. *Gut.* 2004 Dec; 53(12):1878-80. Available at: http://gut.bmj.com/content/53/12/1878.2.full.html

"Autoimmune thyroid disorders and coeliac disease" Collin P, Salmi J, Hällström O, Reunala T, Pasternack A. Autoimmune thyroid disorders and coeliac disease. *Eur J Endocrinol* 1994; 130:137–40. ISSN 0804–4643.

"The presence of the antigliadin antibodies in autoimmune thyroid diseases." Akçay MN, Akçay G. *Hepatogastroenterology.* 2003 Dec; 50 Suppl 2:cclxxix-cclxxx. *PubMed* PMID: 15244201.

"Autoimmune thyroid diseases and coeliac disease." Sategna-Guidetti C, Bruno M, Mazza E, Carlino A, Predebon S, Tagliabue M, Brossa C. *Eur J Gastroenterol. Hepatol.* 1998 Nov; 10(11):927-31. *PubMed* PMID: 9872614.

"Risk factors for and prevalence of thyroid disorders in a cross-sectional study among healthy female relatives of patients with autoimmune thyroid disease." Strieder TG, Prummel MF, Tijssen JG, Endert E, Wiersinga WM. *Clin Endocrinol (Oxf).* 2003 Sep; 59(3):396-401.

"Environmental Exposures and Autoimmune Thyroid Disease." Brent GA. *Thyroid.* 2010; 20(7):755-761.

Chapter 6

Low Dose Naltrexone: http://www.lowdosenaltrexone.org and http://www.ldnresearchtrust.org

"Selenium and the Thyroid Gland." Available at: http://www.medscape.com/viewarticle/777483?pa=1YkwmoR%2BrRbCr1w49YkY7goe%2BFu3fMUssauf%2BEVDlFurylqxMQZ7Tn%2F%2BOyhDuce4VrJxKJt4DRD8mxYr6kYfOw%3D%3D

"Zinc Deficiency Associated with Hypothyroidism: An Overlooked Cause of Severe Alopecia." Ambooken, Betsy. et. al. Available at: https://www.ncbi.nlm.nih.gov/pmc/articles/PMC3746228/

Mackawy AMH, Al-ayed Bushra Mohammed, Al-rashidi Bashayer Mater. "Vitamin D Deficiency and Its Association with Thyroid Disease." *International Journal of Health Sciences.* 2013; 7(3):267-275.

"Medicinal Uses of Seaweed." Ryan Drum. Available at: http://www.eidon.com/MedicinalSeaweeds.pdf

Chapter 7

Sun, Stephanie, et. al. "Validation Of The ReeVue© And Car-
dioCoachCo2© Metabolic Systems For Measuring Resting
Energy Expenditure." *Medicine & Science in Sports &
Exercise*: May 2009 - Volume 41 - Issue 5 - p 42 doi: 10.1249/01.
MSS.0000354690.00049.c8 A-30 Free Communication/
Poster - Exercise Expenditure and Weight Control: MAY 27,
2009

Konrad Kail, N.D., Robert F. Waters, Ph.D., USA. "Managing
Subclinical Hypothyroid Using Resting Metabolic Rate and
Brachioradialis Reflexometry." *Explore!* Volume 17, Number
3, 2008. Available: http://www.nitekmedical.com/files/
EV1732008.pdf

Chapter 8

Muderris II, Boztosun A, Oner G, Bayram F. "Effect of thyroid
hormone replacement therapy on ovarian volume and
androgen hormones in patients with untreated primary
hypothyroidism." *Ann Saudi Med.* 2011 Mar-Apr; 31(2):145-51.

Arner P, Bolinder J, Wennlund A, Ostman J. Influence of thyroid
hormone level on insulin action in human adipose tissue.
Diabetes. 1984 Apr; 33(4):369-75.

Endocr Pract. 2009; 15(3):254-262. © 2009 American Association
of Clinical Endocrinologists. *Journal of Thyroid Research.*
Volume 2011 (2011), Article ID 152850, 9 pages. Available:
http://dx.doi.org/10.4061/2011/152850

Mechanism of Action and Physiologic Effects of Thyroid
Hormones. Available: http://arbl.cvmbs.colostate.edu/
hbooks/pathphys/endocrine/thyroid/physio.html

Rezvani I, DiGeorge AM, Dowshen SA, Bourdony CJ. Action of human growth hormone (hGH) on extrathyroidal conversion of thyroxine (T4) to triiodothyronine (T3) in children with hypopituitarism. *Pediatr Res.* 1981 Jan; 15(1):6-9.

Jørgensen JO, Møller J, Laursen T, Orskov H, Christiansen JS, Weeke J. "Growth hormone administration stimulates energy expenditure and extrathyroidal conversion of thyroxine to triiodothyronine in a dose-dependent manner and suppresses circadian thyrotrophin levels: studies in GH-deficient adults." *Clin Endocrinol* (Oxf). 1994 Nov; 41(5):609-14.

Grunfeld C, Sherman BM, Cavalieri RR. "The acute effects of human growth hormone administration on thyroid function in normal men." *J Clin Endocrinol Metab.* 1988 Nov; 67(5):1111-4.

Root AW, Shulman D, Root J, Diamond F. "The interrelationships of thyroid and growth hormones: effect of growth hormone releasing hormone in hypo- and hyperthyroid male rats." *Acta Endocrinol Suppl* (Copenh). 1986; 279:367-75.

Darras VM, Berghman LR, Vanderpooten A, Kuhn ER. "Growth hormone acutely decreases type III deiodinase in chicken liver." *FEBS Lett* 1992; 310:5-8.

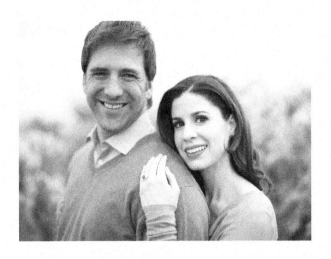

About the Authors

Dr. Robinson and Dr. Bosch have been practicing medicine since 2006. They founded the cutting-edge medical practice, The Hormone Zone©, located in Scottsdale, Arizona.

With their combined passion for Hormone Therapy and Anti-Aging Medicine, their patients have had the benefit of true wellness and optimization. The Hormone Zone© is a uniquely focused specialty practice using a comprehensive approach to hormone balance and treatment, sexual health, and aesthetic medicine. This dynamic couple brings their passion for healthy living and graceful aging to their patients every day. You can find them on an adventure with their three beautiful girls, working on their fitness, or exploring the next healthy restaurant.

CPSIA information can be obtained
at www.ICGtesting.com
Printed in the USA
BVOW03s1020300717
490581BV00003B/4/P